This book is dedicated to all our clients,
who have taught us more over the years
than we could ever teach them.

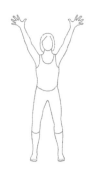

Contents

Foreword

Posture is more than being still and sitting up straight. Posture is found through confidence, moving with grace in your body, and using good biomechanics during work, rest, play, and exercise.

As a chiropractor, I regularly examine posture, range of motion, and the condition of individual vertebra. Posture evaluation allows for a global look at the body: it is a window into the general health of the spine and, more importantly, the master system of the body—the nervous system. When the spine has full range of motion and the nerves are free of interference, the body is able to heal itself from above, down, and inside out.

One of the most common ailments of the 21st century is called Upper Cross Syndrome. Occurring in people who work on a computer or with their hands set out in front of them, this condition is characterized by a forward positioning of the head, a hunching of the shoulders and winging out of the shoulder blades, and a rounding of the upper back. Left uncorrected, this posture can lead to dysfunction and disease affecting the spine and organs.

Sitting all day with bad posture, coupled with maintaining a sedentary lifestyle and eating a standard American diet, is a recipe for degenerative changes in the body and certain health crises. For example, someone may experience chronic tension headaches, caused when the neck muscles overwork to stabilize the spine as the head looks forward and down, or as acute lower back pain caused by sitting, lack of movement, and extremely tight hip flexor muscles.

According to the American Academy of Family Physicians, 9 out of 10 American adults will experience lower back pain; it is the most common reason for lost productivity and missed workdays. This is why many companies are investing in sit-stand workstations and encouraging their employees to walk during breaks. Through movement, vertebral discs are able to bring in nutrients and eliminate waste products. For this reason, movement is essential to a healthy, fully functioning spine and nervous system.

GYROTONIC® Method, Pilates, and yoga are active ways to improve alignment and work on posture. Healthy posture, like many things in life, is a practice that takes time and repetition. You would never put braces on your teeth for one day and expect them to be perfectly straight; likewise, do not expect perfect posture overnight.

This book will provide you with the knowledge and motivation to shift not only your mindset, but also your physical habits. You will instantly become more mindful of your posture as you read this book and follow the simple ways of retraining your body into proper alignment and overall better posture. Lora and Nikki are leaders in their industry, have had tremendous success with thousands of clients, and will provide the guideposts needed to transform your life. As Bruce Lipton, the father of epigenetics has said, "Your genes may load the gun, but your environment pulls the trigger." You are in control of your movement, posture, and lifestyle. This book is the first step to the best version of yourself. I wish you well on this beautiful journey. Namaste.

DR. ELIZABETH M. WISNIEWSKI, DC, CMT, RYT
Vitalistic Visionary, Yoga teacher, Chiropractor

Preface

As children, we run, jump, and play all day. Then we start school, where we spend much of the day sitting at desks. This sedentary lifestyle continues as we become adults who stare at computer screens from 9 to 5, sit in traffic during our commutes, and return home to watch television from our sofas. We have become a society that sits way too much. The result? We've also become a society with a lot of pain, primarily in our backs and necks. In fact, lower back pain is the single leading cause of disability nationwide—experts at the American Academy of Pain Medicine estimate that 60 to 80 percent of the American population will experience a back problem at some point in their life.

As teachers of Pilates, Gyrotonic, and Franklin exercise methods, we spend every day working with clients who struggle with lower back pain and want to move with more ease. We are convinced that the solution to this problem is developing good, natural posture.

Posture is such a fundamental part of having a body that most people don't even notice it. They don't even realize they have bad posture, or how life-changing good posture can be. Having good posture reduces pain, enhances healthy organ function, and helps you become more agile, energetic, and balanced. It doesn't just make you *feel* confident and beautiful, it makes you *look* that way, too, because posture is often one of the first things people notice about you, consciously or not.

It's never too late to fix your posture. In fact, it took both of us many years. After Nikki discovered she had mild scoliosis, she began studying dance and movement regimens, healing arts, energetic body work, and myofascial release. She now lives pain-free. Lora was a professional dancer for over 10 years and suffered from neck and shoulder pain for almost as long. Once she learned how alignment and posture affected these body parts, her pain began to dissolve.

We've come a long way since those painful early days, and you can, too. All you need is a daily practice that maintains your best, natural posture. It doesn't need to be hard or complicated. It just needs to be consistent and frequent.

In this book, we provide exercises to do at home, at work, and on the go to keep you moving with efficient posture throughout your day. You'll discover tools and insights to inspire and strengthen your mind, body, and spirit. You'll learn how posture affects you physically and emotionally, and how to find your own natural posture.

Now take a deep breath, sit up nice and tall, and gently roll your shoulders down and back, letting them melt away from your ears. Exhale.

Let's begin.

Posture Basics

CHAPTER 1

Living Upright

With our technology-driven world and sedentary lifestyles, it's more important than ever to reclaim the design and function of our bodies. Your posture tells a story, probably one about stress, pain, and hours and hours of sitting. By improving your posture, you can rewrite that story and give it a happy ending.

Posture Influences

The human body is meant to move. Not so long ago, we plowed fields and tended crops. Now we sit at desks, in cars, and on couches, staring at screens from sunup to sundown.

The worst part is that the more you sit, the more you want to sit. Bad posture and excessive sitting compress the spine and weaken crucial muscles so that even when you try to stand up and move around, you find yourself fatigued or in pain because you've lost the necessary mobility and strength. Your brain is wired to get better at what you practice, and most of us practice sitting all day every day.

We also practice unhealthy movements that allow us to complete our daily tasks without addressing the underlying problem of posture. If, for example, you're injured, pregnant, or just stiff and weak from too much sitting, your body will compensate for imbalances in ways that affect your posture. Often it will recruit the wrong muscles to do a certain job and end up causing pain and injury.

Your state of mind also influences your posture. What do you do that makes you feel strong and confident? Maybe it's playing a sport or spending time with family and friends. You'll naturally tend to have better posture doing activities you enjoy. When you're down in the dumps, sick, or going through a stressful period, your posture will reflect that as well. Emotional challenges make it harder to align your body and live upright.

The brain is malleable enough to allow you to pick up an instrument or speak another language, so you can learn how to find your best posture and make it your new way of being. You didn't just wake up one day with poor posture; everyday life made it that way. And you can use those same moments in life to create healthy changes.

How Does Posture Affect You?

Healthy, aligned posture lets you sit, stand, and move around without pain, but it also does much more. It improves biological functions throughout your body by increasing circulation, keeping undue pressure off your internal organs, and giving your lungs the room they need to expand. When your body feels better, so does your mind, which is why good posture also promotes confidence and mental clarity.

Poor posture, on the other hand, puts wear and tear on your muscles and joints, leading to unhealthy movement patterns and pain. The resulting fatigue and discomfort affect you mentally and emotionally as well.

Posture and Breathing

Great posture starts with consciously noticing your breath. Do you catch yourself slumped over and holding your breath or taking shallow breaths using your neck and shoulder muscles? That kind of breathing is bad for your posture and your health. When you focus on better breathing techniques, you can dramatically improve your posture and boost your mood. Deep breathing engages the parasympathetic nervous system, which helps you relax and assists in digestion.

The most important muscle related to breathing and posture is the diaphragm. This broad, parachute-shaped muscle attaches to the inner surface of the ribs, separating the upper part of your torso from the lower part. Contracting your diaphragm expands your lungs so they can take in air.

As you do the following breathing exercise, try to sense and imagine your diaphragm and other respiratory muscles in action. Practice three full breaths, and see how it affects your posture.

BREATHING EXERCISE

- Inhale gently through your nose, like you're smelling fresh mountain air. Direct your breath to the front, back, and sides of your diaphragm and rib cage.

- Exhale and make a *haaa* sound like you're fogging a mirror, keeping your neck and jaw relaxed. Feel your abdominal

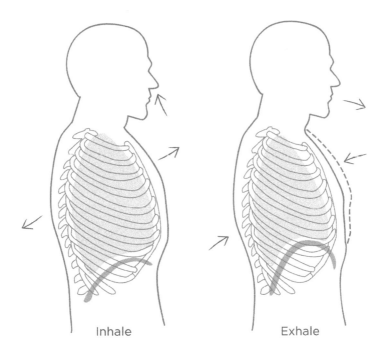

Inhale

Exhale

muscles engage as you draw your ribs together, forcing the air out of your lungs and relaxing the muscles along your spine.

- Inhale and sense your diaphragm flattening out and traveling downward. Feel your ribs expanding to the sides so you can take in more air.

- Exhale as your diaphragm relaxes, expelling the air in your lungs and drawing your ribs closer together.

- Inhale and sense your spine lengthening and decompressing, creating more space between your vertebrae. You should feel taller.

- Exhale and maintain a sense of uprightness. Know that your connection to your breath supports natural posture.

What Good Posture Can Bring to Your Life

Good posture enhances every area of your life. Our culture doesn't support our innate right to natural posture, but with the right techniques, we can regain our ability to sit, stand, work, and play with posture that sustains us and keeps us pain-free. Here are some of the many mental and physical benefits of natural posture.

Protect Yourself from Injury

When you try to perform a certain movement but poor posture has made the necessary muscles too tight or too weak, your body compensates by recruiting other muscles—muscles that aren't in the optimal position to do what you're making them do. You might get injured when, sooner or later, you accidentally force a muscle to do something it's simply not suited for. Efficient posture protects you from these injuries.

Feel and Look Taller

Embody your natural posture, and you'll feel taller. Practice daily, and you'll actually become taller as your spine becomes less crooked and compressed. And when you start to see the positive changes from practicing daily exercises, you'll be inspired to keep it up and see even better results.

Increase Your Confidence

Good posture equals confidence. You're better prepared to take on each day when you carry yourself with ease and without pain. Altering your body language and posture subconsciously influences your thinking and decision making. Get ready for friends and family to notice your new and improved attitude.

Get Stronger

Tension is the enemy of movement. An unbalanced body uses tension instead of strength and flexibility to hold you upright. When your body is aligned, you can move freely, using the correct muscles for each movement instead of recruiting the wrong ones to compensate for weakness. That means any strength training you do will be more effective—and far less likely to cause injuries.

Improve Your Balance

Your sense of balance depends in large part on information that the nerves throughout your body send to your brain via your spinal cord. Good posture keeps your spine long and naturally curved, so those messages can travel freely up and down your spinal cord. Plus it's mechanically easier for your body to stay balanced when it's properly aligned, instead of having a hip jutting out here or a shoulder hunched forward there.

Sleep Better

It's easier to fall asleep and stay asleep when you don't have pain or muscle tightness keeping you awake. The general feeling of relaxation you get from going about your life with natural posture makes a difference as well. Sleeping in a well-aligned position will help you wake up feeling rested and full of energy.

Live without Back Pain

You get good at what you practice, and posture is no exception. Working on good posture will strengthen the muscles and ligaments along your spine so it can easily maintain its natural curves. The more you practice, the better you'll get at it, until you're completely rid of the slouching and poor posture that once made those muscles and ligaments weak and caused you back pain.

Improve Your Athletic Performance

To perform your best at athletic endeavors, you need to be balanced, supported, and focused. Good posture can make that happen. With your lungs working at full capacity and your circulation at its most efficient, you'll benefit from increased stamina. You'll also be able to kick a soccer ball or swing a tennis racket with better form, making you less likely to injure yourself and more likely to perform well.

Your Standing Posture

To fix your posture, you first have to see what's not aligned correctly. Although your posture affects everything you do, most people have no idea what their own posture actually looks like. To remedy that, take two photographs of yourself standing in a neutral position—one from the front and one from the side. Look closely at these photos, and answer the following questions to evaluate the current state of your posture.

- *Where is your head in relation to your torso?* It should be balanced on top of your spine like a golf ball on a tee, with your chin slightly drawn back as you lift through your crown.

- *Do your shoulders round forward?* Your shoulders should be aligned with your earlobes, gently opening your chest.

- *What direction are your palms facing?* Both of your upper arm bones should be turned out with your palms facing up to help align your shoulders and open your chest.

- *Is one shoulder higher than the other?* Your collarbones should be even with each other and balanced over your rib cage.

- **Does your upper back look rounded?** Your sternum and chest should be open with your ribs stacked over your pelvis and under your shoulders.

- **Is your lower back curved or arched?** The top of your pelvis should be aligned vertically with your pubic bone without tilting too far forward or backward.

- **Does your pelvis look even from the front?** The tops of your pelvis bones should be aligned horizontally.

- **Are your knees hyperextended or flexed, or do you appear knock-kneed or bowlegged?** Your legs should be aligned from your hip joint with your knee centered over your second toe.

- **Is your weight evenly distributed over your feet?** You should have equal weight distribution through the tripod formed by your pinky toe, the knuckle of your big toe, and your heel. Your ankles should not be rolling inward or outward.

Your Body Alignment

You already know what incorrect posture feels like, but how would your body feel if it were properly aligned? To find out, stand in a neutral position against a wall. Your head, shoulder blades, and buttocks should be touching the wall, with your heels about two to four inches away from it. From this position, ask yourself the following questions and make the necessary adjustments.

- **What part of your spine is not touching the wall?** Ideal answer: your neck and lower back.

- **How much space is there between your lower back and the wall?** You should have just enough room to place your hand against the wall and slide it behind your lower back. If there's too much room, pull your abs in to close the space. If there's no room, rock your pelvis forward to create a small space (without letting your tummy protrude).

- **Are your knees locked?** Micro-bend your knees (bend them just a tiny bit), and gently engage your thigh muscles until you feel your kneecaps lift a little. You should feel a gentle engagement around your knees without gripping.

- **Do your shoulder blades feel the wall?** They should be able to touch the wall without straining your neck or back.

- **Does the back of your head rest comfortably on the wall?** It should be gently touching the wall.

Now try walking away from the wall while maintaining this alignment. That's how you want your body to be all the time. Implement this posture in your daily activities, and start to subtly change the way you move. Your body will always go back to what it knows best, so you have to keep practicing proper alignment until it becomes your body's default. If you forget how it feels, you can always return to the wall to remind yourself.

CHAPTER 2

What Is Good, Natural Posture?

The answer is different for everyone, and you'll have to explore movement, develop new awareness, and change habits to reach yours. At first it may feel uncomfortable, but finding your natural posture should be just that—natural. If it isn't, it won't work for you.

Posture Myths

You may have been told as a child to stop slouching, stand up straight, or pull your shoulders back. These instructions are well intended, but they don't actually improve your posture. Good posture is dynamic, not static, and supports movement instead of inhibiting it. Let's expose some sneaky myths about posture that may be keeping you in pain.

Myth #1 **It's hard to achieve and maintain good posture.**
Because it's more mechanically efficient, good posture actually takes *less* effort to maintain than bad posture. Yes, it's a
challenge to change patterns you've been stuck in for most of
your life, but you can change any habit with enough awareness
and dedication. Create measurable and realistic goals to slowly
overcome those habits and replace them with better ones. The
better ones will soon feel easier.

Myth #2 **Tucking your pelvis protects your back.**
The natural curves of a neutral spine act like a spring, absorbing force and bearing weight. Tucking your pelvis reverses your
lower back's curve, which makes your spine like a bent spring,
unable to absorb any force efficiently. Without sufficient help
from the spine, your body starts using unfit backup muscles
to complete tasks, and you end up injuring your knees trying
to pick up a heavy object or straining your neck while turning
your head.

Myth #3 **Strong abs equal better posture.**
Developing core strength is trendy right now, but many people
don't fully understand the term "core." They think that if they
have strong abs, they have a strong core. Your core does include
your abdominal muscles, but it also includes your pelvic floor,
diaphragm, certain back muscles, the psoas muscle, and more.
If your abs are strong but your back muscles are weak, your
posture will be inefficient and painful.

Myth #4 **Good posture involves pushing your shoulders
down and back.**
One of the most common overcorrections people make when
trying to fix their posture is to throw their shoulders back and

hold them there. This actually destabilizes your shoulder joints and tenses your neck. Plus, you'll soon get tired and let your shoulders slump again. Once you change your postural habits, your shoulders will sit in the right place without effort.

Myth #5 *Standing up straight shows good posture.*
When you force yourself to stand up straight without awareness of your natural posture, you actually create more tension in your body, not less. Treating your spine like a pillar will only limit your mobility and make you move like a robot. We have curves in our spine to absorb force. Embodying those curves is essential for back health and efficient posture.

Myth #6 *Bad posture is genetic and unchangeable.*
If you believe you're stuck where you are, you will be. If you believe you can work to make a change, you can. Your brain is adaptable enough to learn new movements and habits at any age.

Myth #7 *Slouching isn't that bad for you.*
Sometimes supermodels get paid to slouch in photo spreads, but in everyday life, the effects of bad posture can be serious. The headaches and back pain it commonly causes can be debilitating. In fact, bad posture can negatively affect almost everything, from digestion and circulation to mental health.

Myth #8 *Working in front of a computer is physically easy.*
Sure, you don't have to swing a hammer or move heavy boxes, but if you hunch over a desk all day, your posture is probably in terrible shape. And as you now know, when your posture is unhealthy, your body is unhealthy. Luckily, certain strategies like using a standing desk and taking frequent breaks can let you keep both your desk job and your natural posture.

Myth #9 **Posture has to be held.**

If you have to hold it, it's not sustainable. Your body is designed for movement, and stability comes from balanced, dynamic movement patterns, not from locking yourself into so-called good posture. Being stuck in one position creates tension and unbalanced movement patterns. Efficient posture, on the other hand, lets you move in any direction freely and spontaneously.

Myth #10 **Good posture means never slouching.**

Slouching and flexing are movements you have available to you. You don't want to stay in those positions all the time, but it's good to move through them—it keeps your joints lubricated and mobile. Notice how you're sitting as you read this. Now round forward as deeply as you can, then press through your feet and lengthen your spine. Do that a few times and notice how your resting posture improves.

Walking

Your body needs to move to keep your joints and tissues agile and lubricated. Walking with good posture helps preserve your range of motion so you won't end up shuffling along, hunched over a walker. Looking up and walking with purpose also greatly enhances your alertness and confidence.

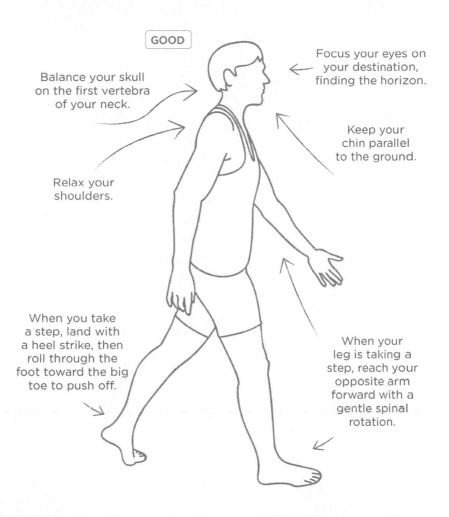

GOOD

Balance your skull on the first vertebra of your neck.

Focus your eyes on your destination, finding the horizon.

Keep your chin parallel to the ground.

Relax your shoulders.

When you take a step, land with a heel strike, then roll through the foot toward the big toe to push off.

When your leg is taking a step, reach your opposite arm forward with a gentle spinal rotation.

Standing

Standing is an active job. It takes stamina and balance to maintain natural posture. It's important to achieve that stamina and balance, because poor standing can cause all sorts of problems. It puts extra wear and tear on your joints and discs, especially your knees and spine, and prevents your muscles from firing the way they're supposed to, making you weaker and more prone to injury.

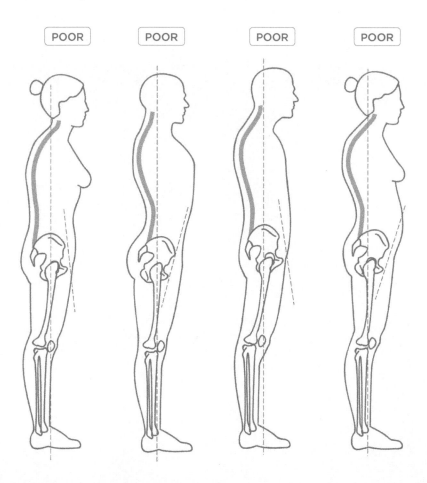

POOR POOR POOR POOR

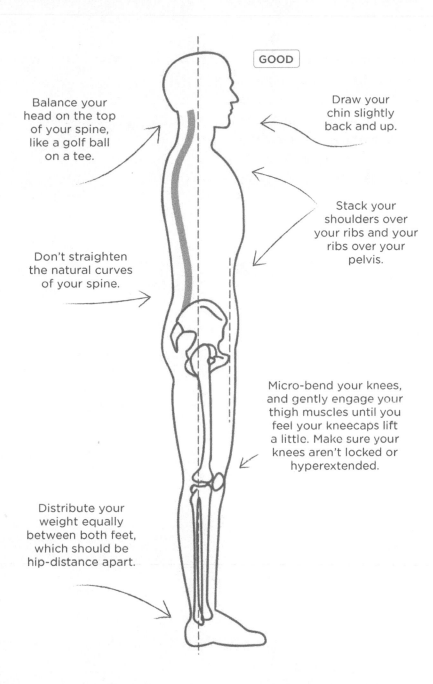

Balance your head on the top of your spine, like a golf ball on a tee.

GOOD

Draw your chin slightly back and up.

Stack your shoulders over your ribs and your ribs over your pelvis.

Don't straighten the natural curves of your spine.

Micro-bend your knees, and gently engage your thigh muscles until you feel your kneecaps lift a little. Make sure your knees aren't locked or hyperextended.

Distribute your weight equally between both feet, which should be hip-distance apart.

Sitting

Many experts agree that the longer you sit, the more likely you are to develop diabetes, heart disease, and other ailments, and potentially die prematurely—even with regular exercise. This means you need to kick the habit of sitting and begin to move. And when you do sit, use these postural tips.

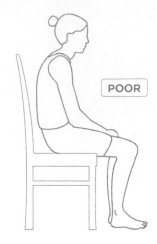

POOR

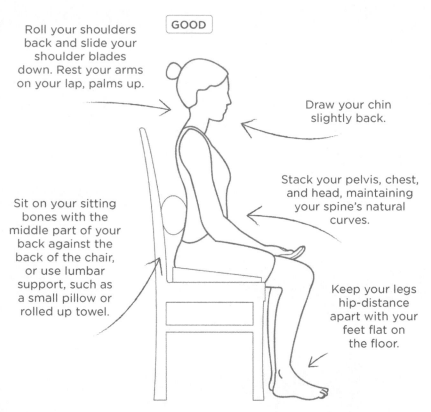

GOOD

Roll your shoulders back and slide your shoulder blades down. Rest your arms on your lap, palms up.

Draw your chin slightly back.

Stack your pelvis, chest, and head, maintaining your spine's natural curves.

Sit on your sitting bones with the middle part of your back against the back of the chair, or use lumbar support, such as a small pillow or rolled up towel.

Keep your legs hip-distance apart with your feet flat on the floor.

Working at a Desk

Working at a desk for long hours takes a toll on your body. Without proper posture and ergonomics, you're likely to suffer from headaches, neck and back pain, tight hip flexors and hamstrings, and general stiffness. Make sure you're working with good posture, and you'll have a more productive day.

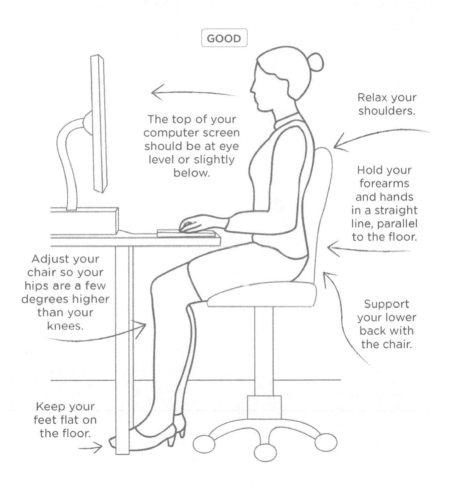

GOOD

The top of your computer screen should be at eye level or slightly below.

Relax your shoulders.

Hold your forearms and hands in a straight line, parallel to the floor.

Adjust your chair so your hips are a few degrees higher than your knees.

Support your lower back with the chair.

Keep your feet flat on the floor.

Driving

If you're like most Americans, you spend a lot of time in your car. Unfortunately, it's easy to have bad posture while driving. Using only one hand on the wheel creates unbalanced shoulders and ribs, slouching dumps pressure into your back and legs, and craning your head forward to see the road causes tension in your neck. On your next drive, take these pointers with you.

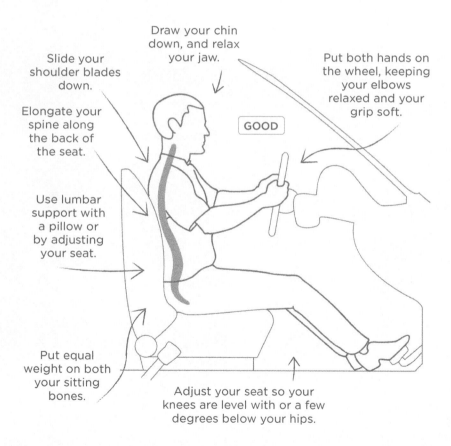

Draw your chin down, and relax your jaw.

Slide your shoulder blades down.

Put both hands on the wheel, keeping your elbows relaxed and your grip soft.

Elongate your spine along the back of the seat.

GOOD

Use lumbar support with a pillow or by adjusting your seat.

Put equal weight on both your sitting bones.

Adjust your seat so your knees are level with or a few degrees below your hips.

Sleeping

You sleep without much conscious control of your body, which means you can end up twisting your spine, tucking your pelvis, and otherwise throwing off your posture without even realizing it. Sleeping on your stomach is especially bad for you because it pulls your neck out of alignment. Train your body to sleep in a healthier position with these techniques.

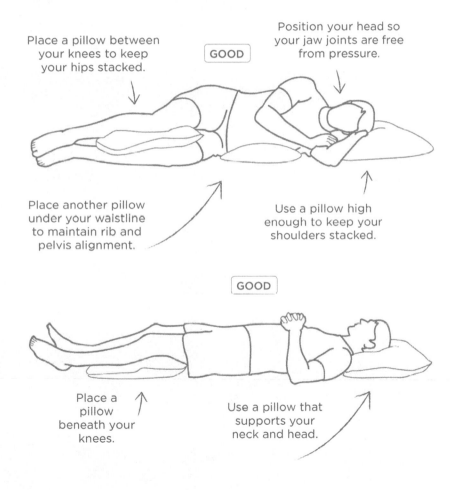

Place a pillow between your knees to keep your hips stacked.

GOOD

Position your head so your jaw joints are free from pressure.

Place another pillow under your waistline to maintain rib and pelvis alignment.

Use a pillow high enough to keep your shoulders stacked.

GOOD

Place a pillow beneath your knees.

Use a pillow that supports your neck and head.

Lifting

Proper lifting techniques are essential for preventing injuries to your muscles, joints, and spinal discs. Avoid leaning over from your waist, tucking your pelvis, and reaching with your shoulders. Never lift and twist at the same time—the simultaneous spinal bend and rotation creates compression and disc injuries. Instead, follow these guidelines for a healthy lift.

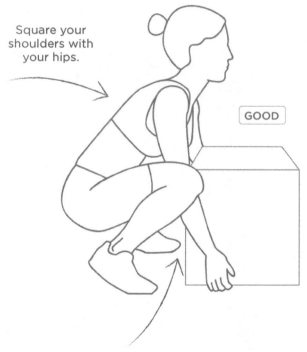

Square your shoulders with your hips.

GOOD

Squat in front of the object by bending your knees, not your back.

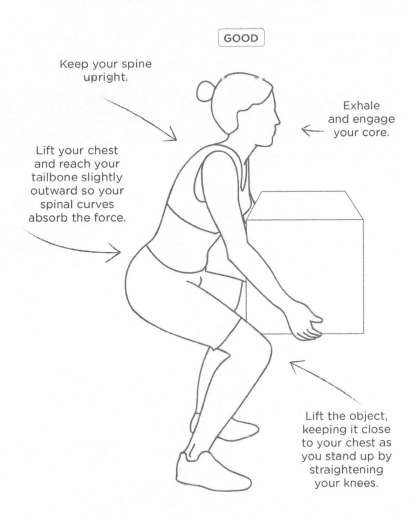

GOOD

Keep your spine upright.

Exhale and engage your core.

Lift your chest and reach your tailbone slightly outward so your spinal curves absorb the force.

Lift the object, keeping it close to your chest as you stand up by straightening your knees.

Reading

Curling up with a book is good for your mind, but it can be hard on your body. Whether you're reading a paperback or on a tablet device, it can be difficult to concentrate on the words in front of you if you're in discomfort or pain. These guidelines will make reading easier on your neck, shoulders, and back.

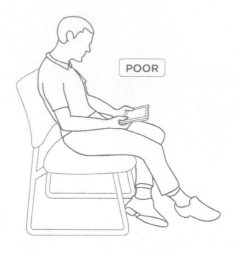

POOR

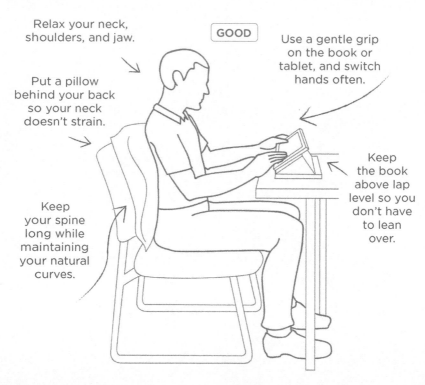

Relax your neck, shoulders, and jaw.

GOOD

Use a gentle grip on the book or tablet, and switch hands often.

Put a pillow behind your back so your neck doesn't strain.

Keep the book above lap level so you don't have to lean over.

Keep your spine long while maintaining your natural curves.

Texting

Texting makes it easy to connect with people but difficult to maintain natural posture. Your head weighs about 10 pounds, which means that for every inch your head is off its central axis, your spine experiences 10 extra pounds of pressure. This can cause disc injuries, spinal nerve compression, and more.

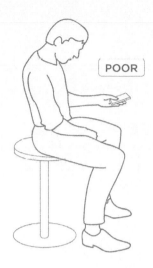

POOR

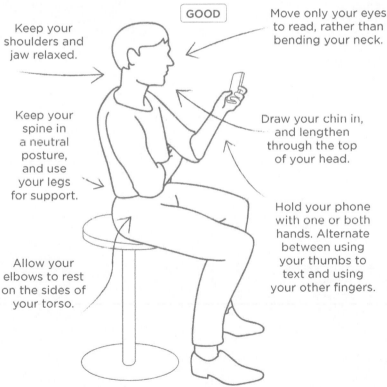

GOOD

Keep your shoulders and jaw relaxed.

Move only your eyes to read, rather than bending your neck.

Keep your spine in a neutral posture, and use your legs for support.

Draw your chin in, and lengthen through the top of your head.

Hold your phone with one or both hands. Alternate between using your thumbs to text and using your other fingers.

Allow your elbows to rest on the sides of your torso.

Carrying

Do you end your day with sore shoulders because of all the stuff you're always lugging around? Heavy bags and purses can strain your neck and shoulders and pull your spine out of alignment. Set your bags down whenever you can, and give your shoulders a break by using a roller bag or backpack. When that's not possible, keep these tips in mind.

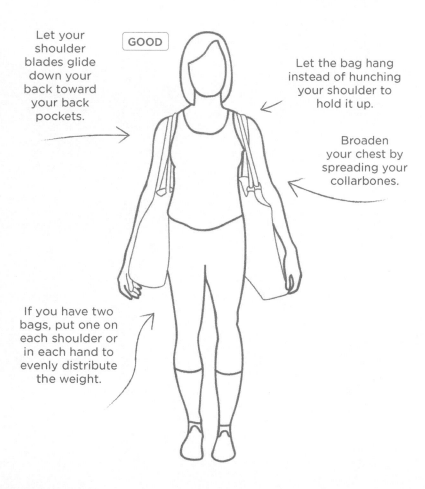

Let your shoulder blades glide down your back toward your back pockets.

GOOD

Let the bag hang instead of hunching your shoulder to hold it up.

Broaden your chest by spreading your collarbones.

If you have two bags, put one on each shoulder or in each hand to evenly distribute the weight.

Gardening

Hobbies like gardening, crafting, and sewing are all done in positions that can be tough on your neck, shoulders, back, and knees. You might notice joint pain or achy muscles after a long session of knitting or weeding. But with a little practice and awareness, you can enjoy your hobby pain-free.

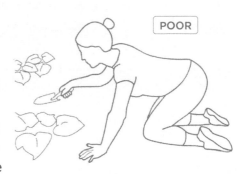

POOR

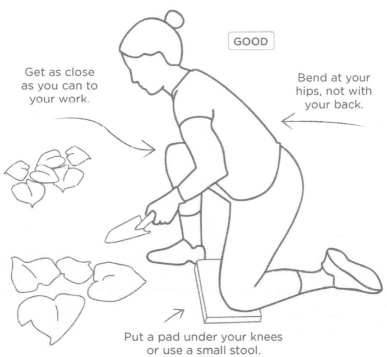

GOOD

Get as close as you can to your work.

Bend at your hips, not with your back.

Put a pad under your knees or use a small stool.

Pregnancy

Between the extra weight and the pressure on your abdominal cavity, pregnancy is a big challenge to postural alignment. It's easy to unconsciously compensate by hyperextending your knees and lower back. On top of that, your diaphragm has less room to expand, which inhibits breathing and relaxation. Keep the following tips in mind for better pregnancy posture.

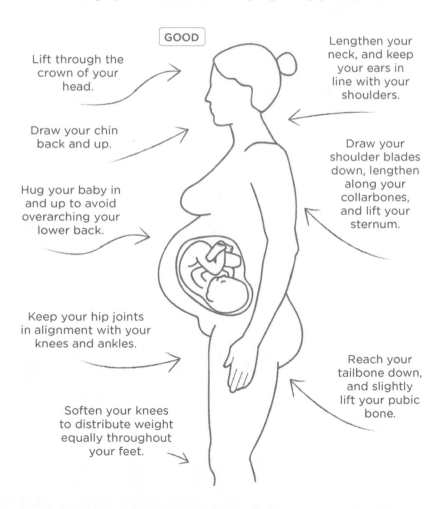

GOOD

Lift through the crown of your head.

Draw your chin back and up.

Hug your baby in and up to avoid overarching your lower back.

Keep your hip joints in alignment with your knees and ankles.

Soften your knees to distribute weight equally throughout your feet.

Lengthen your neck, and keep your ears in line with your shoulders.

Draw your shoulder blades down, lengthen along your collarbones, and lift your sternum.

Reach your tailbone down, and slightly lift your pubic bone.

Daily Posture Exercises & Routines

Getting Started

Now that you've learned the proper way to sit, stand, walk, and carry, we'll introduce you to postural exercises that you can practice throughout your day. Most of the exercises use props that you can easily access, like a wall or a chair. We also incorporate resistance bands, and floor mats to help support you. Here are a few helpful tips:

- *Buy a Variety of Resistance Bands.* Usually made of latex, they look like wide ribbons. (If you are allergic, use latex-free bands.) They are often color-coded according to tension. It's good to have options for at least three different levels of resistance.

- *Choose an Exercise Mat.* Yoga mats are normally thinner, while Pilates mats tend to be thicker. If you want more cushioning for your hips and back, opt for the latter. If you are traveling and don't have a mat handy, you can lay a couple towels on the ground for cushioning.

- *Exercise at Your Own Pace.* You know your body best. Relax your body when you are exercising and initiate movements that feel comfortable for you. Avoid any movements that trigger pain.

- *Watch our Exercise Videos.* We've made companion videos to demonstrate some of the exercises in this book. You can find them at www.PainFreePostureHandbook.com or on our YouTube channel: Pain-Free Posture Handbook.

Anatomically Speaking

In the exercises, we use certain terminology to refer to parts of the body. Reference this chart to get familiar with your anatomy as you practice the posture exercises and experience results.

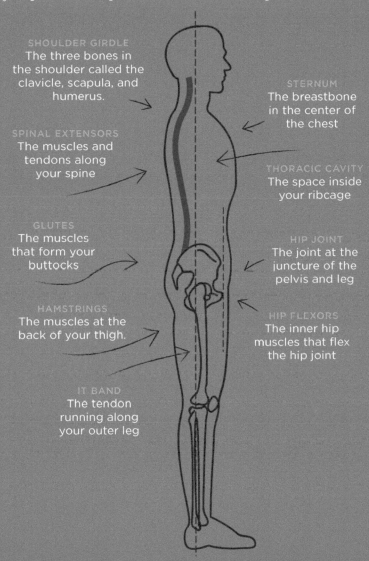

SHOULDER GIRDLE
The three bones in the shoulder called the clavicle, scapula, and humerus.

SPINAL EXTENSORS
The muscles and tendons along your spine

GLUTES
The muscles that form your buttocks

HAMSTRINGS
The muscles at the back of your thigh.

IT BAND
The tendon running along your outer leg

STERNUM
The breastbone in the center of the chest

THORACIC CAVITY
The space inside your ribcage

HIP JOINT
The joint at the juncture of the pelvis and leg

HIP FLEXORS
The inner hip muscles that flex the hip joint

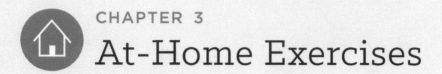

CHAPTER 3

At-Home Exercises

You can work on your natural posture even during everyday tasks like brushing your teeth or standing at your kitchen counter. Explore these mindful movement sequences in the comfort of your own home throughout your day, and notice how much your posture begins to improve.

Wake-Up Stretch

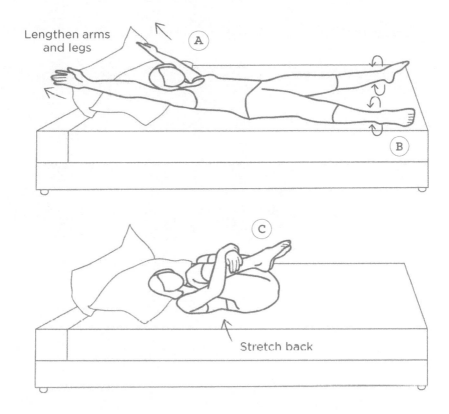

Lengthen arms and legs

A

B

C

Stretch back

EFFECTS Stimulates your nervous system, lubricates your joints, gets your blood flowing. EQUIPMENT A bed.

1 When you wake up, take three deep breaths and visualize moving through your day with ease. Stretch your arms and legs away from each other in a big X, (A) and circle your wrists and ankles. (B)

2 Hug your knees into your chest, (C) and stretch your back. ▶

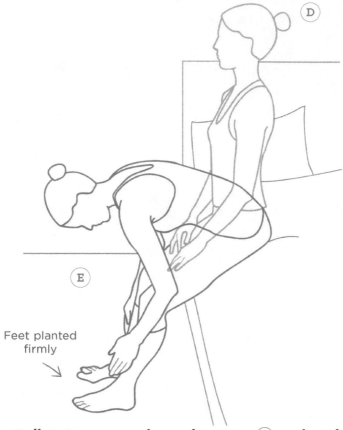

Feet planted
firmly

3 Roll up into a neutral seated position Ⓓ on the side of your
   bed with your feet flat on the floor.

4 Using both hands, gently perform a series of taps down the
   front, back, and sides of your legs to your feet, Ⓔ then tap
   back up to your chest and shoulders and brush your fingers
   down your arms.

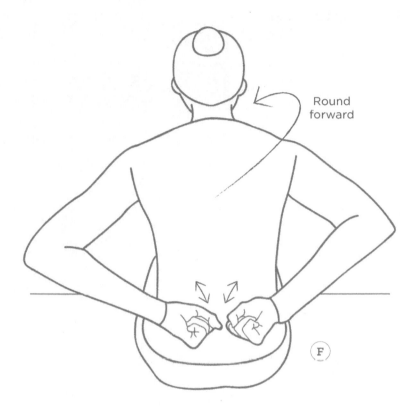

Round
forward

F

5　Round forward and gently pound both sides of your lower
　back with a soft fist. (F)

6　Elongate your back and return to neutral seated position, (D)
　noticing your effortlessly natural posture.

> **TIP:** Set your alarm five minutes early so you'll have time
> to start your day with this stretch.

Two-Minute Toothbrush Warm-Up

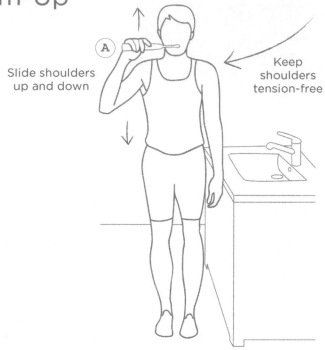

Slide shoulders up and down

A

Keep shoulders tension-free

EFFECTS Strengthens your calves and ankles, aligns your shoulders, improves your balance. EQUIPMENT A toothbrush, ideally an electric one with a two-minute timer.

1 Visualize a cord attached to the top of your head, pulling your crown toward the ceiling and aligning your head, shoulders, chest, and pelvis over your legs.

2 Start your toothbrush.

3 For one minute, slide your shoulders up and down, as if polishing the back of your rib cage. (A) Finish with your shoulders melting away from your ears.

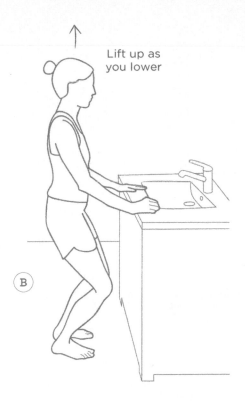

Lift up as
you lower

B

4 For the second minute, use one hand to stabilize yourself as you lift and lower your heels, performing calf raises while maintaining alignment. Test your balance by taking your hand off the counter.

5 When your toothbrush stops (or two minutes have passed), finish by bending your knees (B) to stretch your Achilles tendons and calf muscles.

TIPS: Don't tense your shoulders during step 3 or roll your ankles in or out during the calf raises in step 4. Make sure to micro-bend your knees to avoid hyperextension. Avoid this exercise if you have acute Achilles tendon or calf injuries.

Shower Stretch

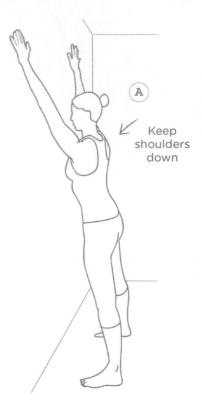

Keep
shoulders
down

EFFECTS Decompresses and articulates your spine, stretches your hamstrings. EQUIPMENT A shower or wall.

1 With the water running, stand facing away from the shower head and looking toward the wall in front of you.

2 Slide your hands up the wall as your shoulder blades slide down. (A) Keeping your shoulders down, reach a little farther up with your hands, drawing your ribs away from your pelvis. Take three deep breaths as you decompress your spine.

3 Keeping the length in your spine, step away from the wall (B) and stand facing away from the showerhead so the warm water is flowing down your back.

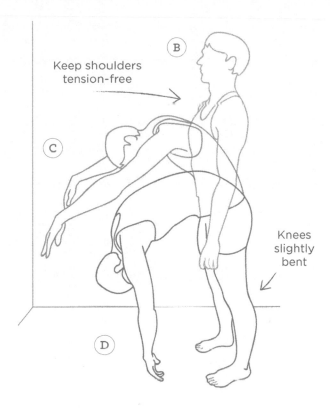

Keep shoulders
tension-free

Knees
slightly
bent

4   Begin to slowly roll your spine forward one vertebra at a
     time. (c) Nod your chin to your chest, soften your sternum,
     and curl over your heart, ribs, and belly button. With your
     knees slightly bent, reach gently toward your feet, stretching
     your hamstrings. (D)

5   Take a deep breath and visualize your back filling up with air
     like a parachute.

6   Pushing down through your legs, slowly roll back up through
     your spine to a standing position. (B)

Pelvic Clock

TIPS: Move slowly without tension, and breathe. Initiate the movement from your pelvis. Stabilize your legs and hips, and keep hip flexors and glutes relaxed. Avoid this exercise if you have acute back pain.

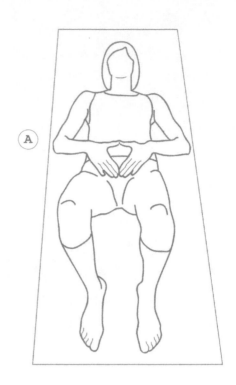

EFFECTS Helps you find and maintain the integrity of your spinal curves, warms up your lower back and pelvic floor muscles, enhances pelvic mobility. **EQUIPMENT** A mat and a pillow or towel (optional).

1 Lie on your back with your knees bent, your feet flat on the floor, and your arms by your sides. Use a pillow under your neck or lower back for support if needed. Your lower back should have a soft, natural arch. (Imagine a few ladybugs being able to crawl through.)

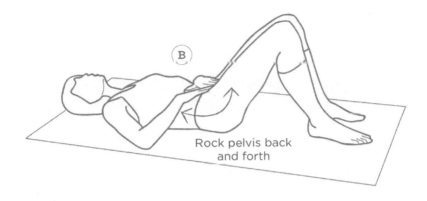

Rock pelvis back
and forth

2   Place your hands on your pelvis, reaching your fingers
    toward your pubic bone and your thumbs toward your belly
    button. (A) The triangle of your hands should be horizontally
    level. Imagine resting a drink on your lower abs and not
    spilling it. Your ribs should be softening down toward your
    belly button and anchoring you into the ground. This is the
    neutral position.

3   With your hands still in the triangle, create an arch by
    rocking your pelvis toward your fingers/pubic bone. (B) The
    move is very small. Then rock back toward your thumbs/
    belly button. Rock back and forth eight times, breathing
    naturally. Finish in neutral. Notice how your back feels.

4   Next, imagine a clock face on your pelvis. Trace a circle with
    your pelvis, connecting all the numbers from 1 through 12.
    Feel your back stretching and lengthening.

Kitchen Counter Stretch

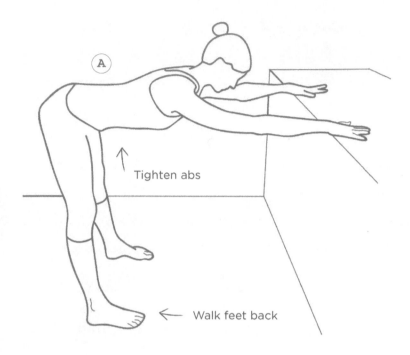

Tighten abs

← Walk feet back

EFFECTS Stretches your hip flexors and hamstrings, increases your hip mobility, extends your spine.
EQUIPMENT A kitchen counter.

1 In a standing position, place both hands on the counter in front of you, shoulder-distance apart.

2 Walk your feet back as you fold forward from your hips so that your body forms an upside-down L, with your chest and head slightly above your shoulders in a line with your spine. (A) Keep your spine elongated and engage your core.

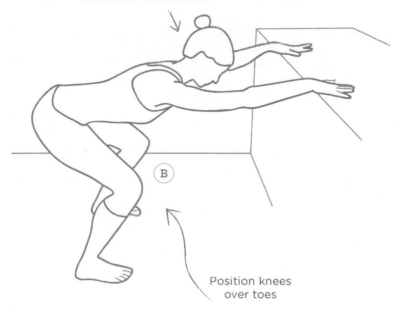

Keep head and chest
lifted above shoulders

B

Position knees
over toes

3　Keeping your knees aligned over your big toes, inhale as
you bend your knees Ⓑ and exhale as you straighten them.
Repeat five times. ▶

TIPS: Don't drop your chest and head below your shoulders or hyperextend your knees, and don't forget to use your core. Avoid this exercise if you have shoulder and hip injuries.

Kitchen Counter Stretch *continued*

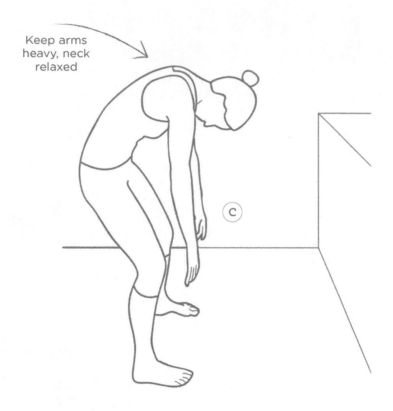

Keep arms
heavy, neck
relaxed

4 Soften your knees, remove your hands from the counter, ⓒ and slowly roll back up.

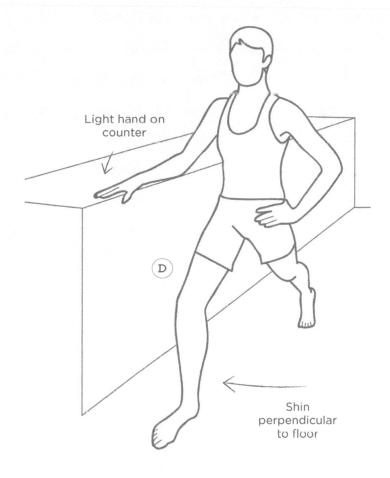

Light hand on
counter

D

Shin
perpendicular
to floor

5 With your right hand on the counter for balance, turn
to the side. Step forward into a lunge with your right leg.
Keeping your right knee bent, reach through your left heel
while keeping your left leg as straight as possible. (D) ▸

Kitchen Counter Stretch *continued*

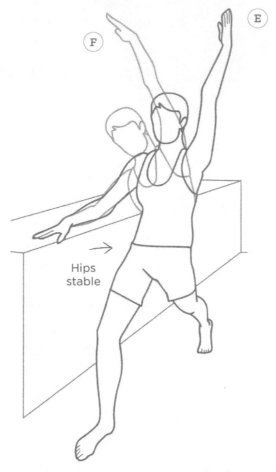

6 Reach your left arm up toward the ceiling, (E) pulling in your abs and pushing your outside hip forward so that it's square with your inside hip and shoulders. Try reaching toward the counter for an extra side stretch (optional). (F)

7 Hold for five deep breaths.

8 Repeat steps 5 through 7 on the other side.

Cat-Cow, Bird Dog Sequence

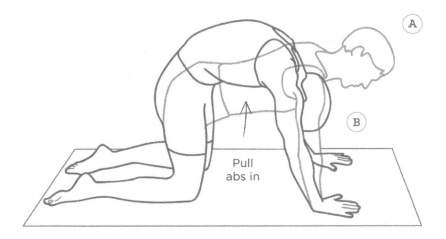

Pull
abs in

EFFECTS Improves your balance, coordination, and sense of where you are in space; strengthens your spine and core.

EQUIPMENT A mat.

1   Get down on your hands and knees on a mat, with your wrists directly under your shoulders and your knees directly below your hips. (A) This is the neutral position.

2   Pointing your nose toward your pubic bone, round your spine upward like a cat arching its back. (B) (This is the "cat" portion of the cat-cow.) ▶

Cat-Cow, Bird Dog Sequence *continued*

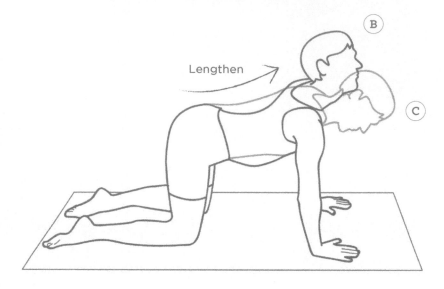

Lengthen

3 Now stretch your spine in the opposite direction, arching it toward the floor as you reach the crown of your head toward your tailbone. (B) Soften your elbows. (This is the "cow" portion of the cat-cow.)

4 Return to a relaxed all-fours position with your spine neutral like a table. (C) Spread your fingers and distribute your weight evenly over your hands. Press the floor away as you engage your back and chest muscles to stabilize your shoulders.

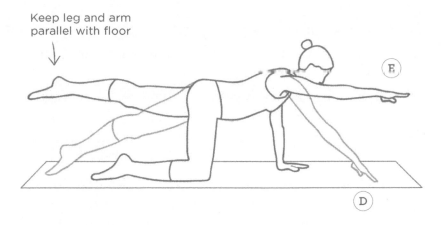

Keep leg and arm
parallel with floor

E

D

5 Inhale and straighten your right arm out forward and your
left leg out backward until they're touching the floor with
just the fingertips and toes. (D)

6 Exhale, and, using your core, lift your right arm and left leg
straight up in a line with your hip and shoulder joints, until
they're parallel with the floor. (E) (This is the "bird dog,"
because it makes you look like an alert hunting dog.)

7 Repeat steps 4 through 6 using your left arm and right leg.

8 Perform three sets of the whole sequence, from cat-cow to
bird dog.

TIPS: During the bird dog, keep your head, arm, and leg
aligned with your spine. Engage your core so your lower
back doesn't arch. Avoid this sequence if you have knee
or wrist injuries.

Supine Hamstring Stretch

EFFECTS Increases your hip mobility, stretches your hamstrings and IT band. EQUIPMENT A mat and a medium-to-heavy resistance band.

1   Lying on your back on a mat, bend your right knee toward your chest and place a resistance band around the sole of your right foot, holding the band with both hands. Your left leg can be bent or straight, whichever is more comfortable.

2   Extend your right leg so that it forms a 45- to 90-degree angle with the ground. (A) (Micro-bend your knee if you have tight hamstrings.) Lengthen through the crown of your head.

3   Initiating the movement with your hip joint, move your leg in a smooth, clockwise circle with the support of the band, as if your leg was tracing a circle on the ceiling. (B) Repeat six times.

4   Repeat step 3, this time going counterclockwise.

5   When you're finished with the circles, straighten that leg and bring it slowly across your midline to stretch your IT band (the tendon running along your outer leg). Don't let any part of your pelvis come up off the floor.

6   Repeat the whole sequence with your left leg.

> TIPS: If you can't keep a straight leg, maintain a micro-bend in your knee. Keep an easy grip on the resistance band. Shoulders and hips should be relaxed and on the mat. Avoid this exercise if you have a hamstring injury or acute sciatic-nerve pain.

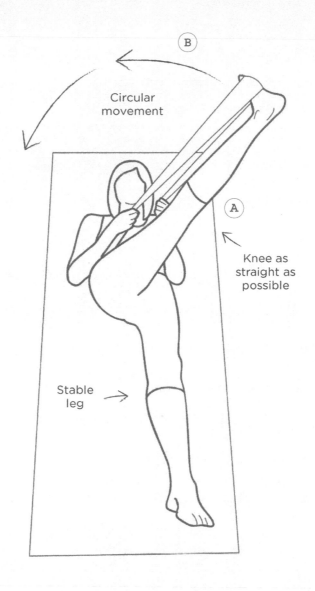

B

Circular
movement

A

Knee as
straight as
possible

Stable
leg

Clam Sequence

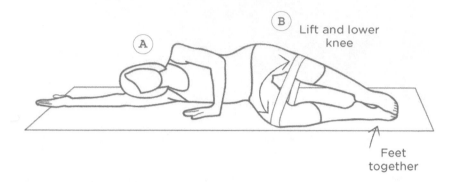

B Lift and lower knee

A

Feet together

EFFECTS Strengthens your glutes, increases pelvic stability.
EQUIPMENT A light-to-medium resistance band, a mat, and
a pillow (optional).

1 Lie on your side and tie the resistance band around your
   knees in a fairly tight knot, making sure your hips are
   stacked on top of each other. Rest your head on your arm
   or a pillow. (A)

2 Keeping your pelvis still and your feet together, lift and
   lower your top knee (B) as if your legs were a clamshell
   opening and closing. Repeat 10 times.

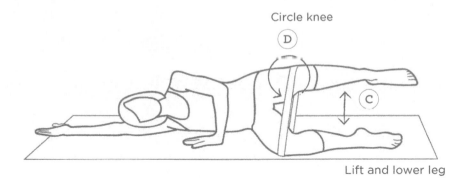

Circle knee

Lift and lower leg

3 Next, lift and lower your entire leg from the hip, as if opening the page of a book. (c) (This move is sometimes called a
   "fire hydrant" because it makes you look like a dog lifting its
   leg!) Repeat 10 times.

4 Hold your leg up at hip height, and draw a small circle
   with your knee. (D) Repeat 10 times clockwise and 10 times
   counterclockwise.

5 Repeat on your other side.

> **TIPS:** Use your glutes. Keep your hips square to avoid
> your top hip rolling forward.

Indoor Swim

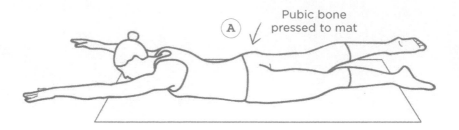

A Pubic bone pressed to mat

EFFECTS Strengthens your lower back, spinal extensors, glutes, and hamstrings; opens up your chest muscles.
EQUIPMENT A mat.

1 Lie face-down on the mat with your legs hip-distance apart. Reach your arms and legs away from your center, making sure your abs are drawing up and away from the floor and your pubic bone is gently pressing down to support your lower back. (A) Engage your glutes.

2 Lift your left arm up, (B) then bring it back down. Repeat with your right arm.

3 Lift your left leg up, then bring it back down. Repeat with your right leg. (C)

4 Now, with your head gently floating a couple inches above the floor, reach your left arm and right leg up at the same time. (B) (C) Repeat using your right arm and left leg.

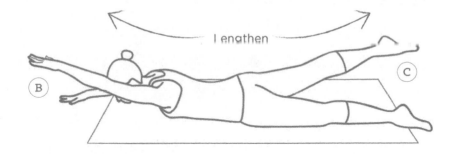

5   Switch between the two sides as if you were swimming, lifting your left arm and right leg as you lower your right arm and left leg. Breathe naturally and keep your abs engaged.

6   Finish by resting in child's pose to stretch your lower back: Remaining face down, sit on your heels, and relax your arms at your sides.

TIPS: This exercise is about lengthening your spine so don't worry about how high you lift your arms and legs. Focusing your eyes toward the floor will help you keep a straight line with your back.

Spinal Roll-Up

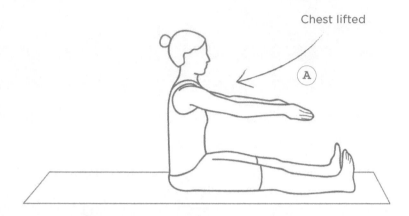

Chest lifted

A

EFFECTS Articulates your spine, strengthens your core.
EQUIPMENT A mat.

1 Sit on the mat with your legs out in front of you, straight or slightly bent. Reach your arms straight out in front of you as well. (A)

2 Exhale, tilt your pelvis back, and gradually lower your spine onto the mat, (B) one vertebra at a time, until your shoulders and head reach the mat.

3 Inhale and bring your arms overhead, (C) stretching them toward the wall behind you.

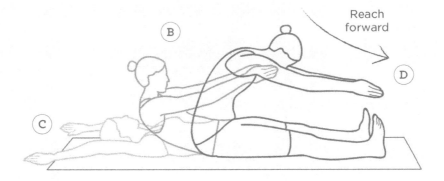

Reach forward

4 Exhale and reach your arms toward your toes. Nod your head forward, and roll up to a seated position one vertebra at a time. Continue rolling toward your toes, finishing in your deepest stretch. (D)

5 Repeat five times.

TIPS: Articulate your spine one vertebra at a time. Make the move slow and deliberate without relying on momentum. Remember to breathe. For a slightly easier version, place your feet under a couch for support or use a resistance band to assist in the roll-up.

Pelvic Curl Sequence

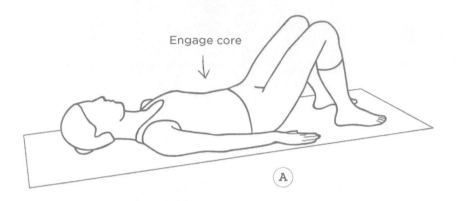

Engage core

(A)

EFFECTS Strengthens your hamstrings, glutes, and spinal extensors. EQUIPMENT A mat.

1 Lie on your back with your knees bent, your arms alongside your body, and your feet flat on the floor in line with your hips. (A)

2 Inhale and imagine your spine as a string of pearls. As you exhale, start to peel it off the mat from your tailbone, one pearl at a time, (B) until you get to your rib cage.

3 Inhale and hold for a moment. As you exhale, slowly articulate your spine back down one vertebra at a time until you relax into your neutral starting position. (A)

4 Repeat this pelvic curl five times.

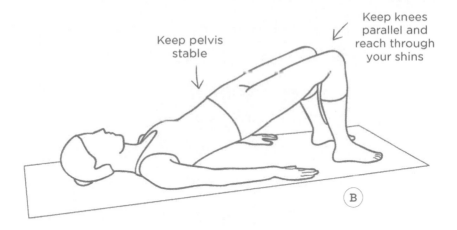

Keep pelvis
stable

Keep knees
parallel and
reach through
your shins

B

5 Now inhale from your neutral position, and as you exhale, lift your spine up into a diagonal line in one movement. (B) Make sure your abs and glutes are engaged.

6 Inhale and lower your pelvis back down to neutral.

7 Repeat this bridge 10 times.

8 On the last bridge, keep your pelvis up and do 10 pulses— small thrusts that only lift and lower your pelvis a tiny bit.

TIPS: At the high point, your pelvis should form a straight line with your knees and chest. Engage your core. Avoid this exercise if you have acute back pain or if you don't have a mat or padded surface to do it on.

Tennis Ball Foot Massage

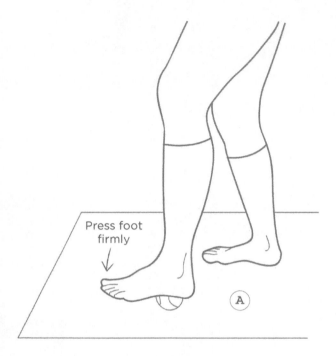

Press foot
firmly

(A)

EFFECTS Stretches and massages your feet.
EQUIPMENT A tennis ball.

1 Stand in a neutral position, taking notice of both your feet.

2 Step onto a tennis ball with your left foot, bending your
   knees and pressing the ball firmly into the sole of your foot.
   (A) Roll it against the center and sides of your foot, maintaining that firm pressure the whole time.

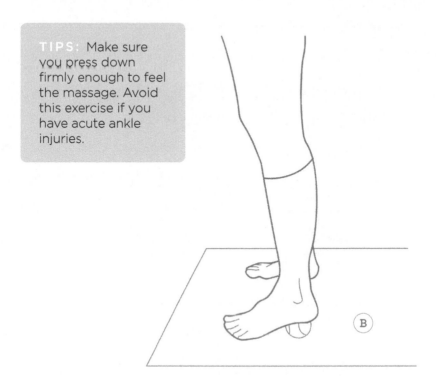

TIPS: Make sure you press down firmly enough to feel the massage. Avoid this exercise if you have acute ankle injuries.

3 Finish with the ball under your heel, (B) straightening your leg to provide more pressure.

4 Step off the ball and notice how your left foot feels in comparison to your right foot.

5 Repeat with your right foot.

Upper-Body Floor Twist

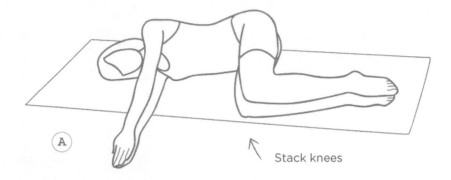

(A)

↖ Stack knees

EFFECTS Rotates your spine, stretches your shoulders and chest. EQUIPMENT A mat.

1　Lie on your side on a mat with your knees bent at a 90-degree angle and both arms reaching straight out in front of you. (A) Your knees should be stacked on top of each other, as should your shoulders.

2　Inhale and use your top arm to slowly trace an arc on the floor over your head. (B) Your arm should stay straight, and your fingers should never leave the floor (unless it hurts your shoulder to keep them there). Keep your knees in place as your chest opens up and your spine rotates toward the floor.

3　Exhale, ending the motion with both hands reaching away from each other in a wide T, (C) stretching your chest and spine. Your knees should not move at all.

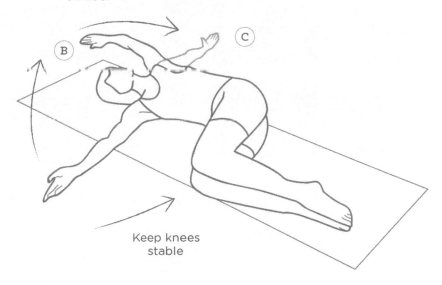

Trace arc with fingers
on floor

B

C

Keep knees
stable

4 Staying on the same side, reverse the movement, tracing the arc over your head the opposite way and ending in your original side-stacked position. Repeat the whole sequence three times.

5 Roll over and lay on the other side of your body. Repeat steps 1 through 4.

TIPS: Engage your core, without holding your breath. Avoid this exercise if you have shoulder or spine injuries.

Shoulder-Stretching Sequence

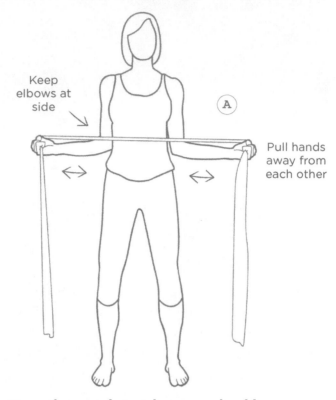

Keep elbows at side

A

Pull hands away from each other

EFFECTS Strengthens and stretches your shoulders.
EQUIPMENT A light-to-medium resistance band.

1 Start by shrugging your shoulders in a circular motion, five times forward and five times backward.

2 With your elbows at your sides, arms bent at a 90-degree angle, and your palms up, hold the resistance band with both hands. Keeping your elbows glued to your sides, pull your hands away from each other and rotate your shoulders outward against the resistance of the band. (A) Repeat 10 to 15 times.

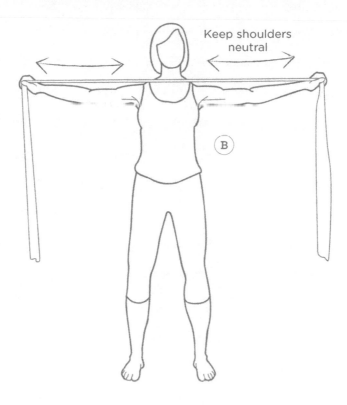

Keep shoulders neutral

B

3   Now do the same thing but with your palms down and your arms straight out in front of you at shoulder height. Draw your hands away from each other, rotating your shoulders outward against the resistance of the band, until your arms are all the way out to your sides and your body forms a T. (B) Repeat 10 to 15 times.

TIPS: You can do this exercise sitting or standing. Keep your shoulders neutral so they stay mobile, and don't let tension pull them up. Avoid this exercise if you have shoulder injuries or pain.

Arm-Toning Sequence

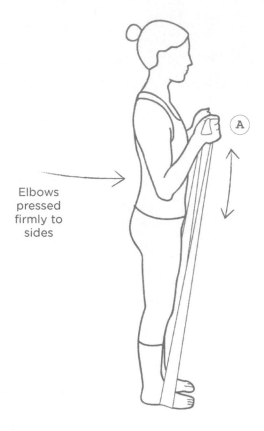

Elbows
pressed
firmly to
sides

EFFECTS Tones your arms, helps you practice your posture.
EQUIPMENT A resistance band (lighter is better).

1 Stand on the middle of the resistance band, and hold one
end in each hand. With your posture neutral and your
elbows glued to your sides, draw your hands, palms facing
each other, toward your shoulders, as if doing bicep curls
with handheld weights. (A) Repeat 15 times.

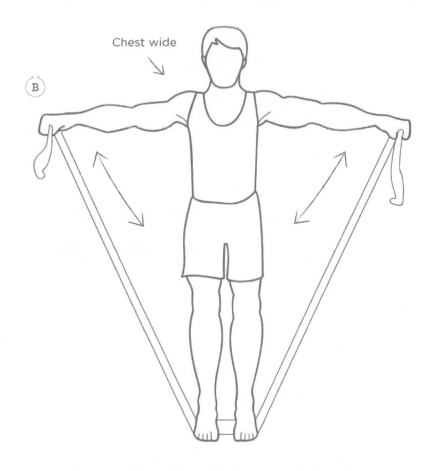

Chest wide

B

2 Now hold the ends of the resistance band with your palms down, and open your arms straight out to the sides until your body forms a T. (B) Repeat 15 times.

3 Next, pull the ends of the resistance band straight out behind you, keeping your elbows straight and moving from your shoulders. Repeat 15 times. ▶

Arm-Toning Sequence *continued*

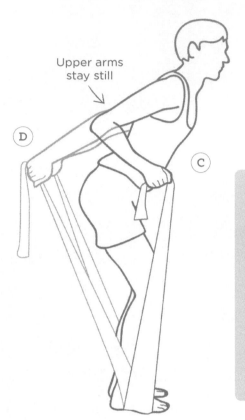

Upper arms
stay still

D

C

TIPS: Keep your shoulders neutral, and don't let tension pull them up. Be careful not to grip the resistance band too tightly. Stay relaxed and fluid. Avoid this exercise if you have acute shoulder or wrist pain.

4   Finally, lean forward from your hips and bend your elbows at 90 degrees. (C) Pull the ends of the resistance band straight out behind you. (D) Your upper arm should stay completely still as you pull by straightening your elbows. Repeat 15 times.

CHAPTER 4

At-Work Exercises

Why not make the most of your day by working on your natural posture as you work at your job? Improve your workstation's ergonomics. Use a standing desk or set a timer to remind yourself to stand up every half hour, and practice these office-compatible exercises to sustain healthy posture at work.

Snow Angels

EFFECTS Centers your energy, increases your awareness of your body. EQUIPMENT A chair (optional).

The body has four sides: front, back, right, and left. In the GYROTONIC® Method, the center of these four sides is called the "fifth line" and it's considered an energetic center point.

1 Start in a standing position or sitting in a chair with a neutral spine.

2 Reach your arms down along your sides with your palms facing forward. (A) Imagine the fifth line of your arm and of each finger as you reach your arms out long. Sense the fifth line of your legs as you press down with them and the fifth line of your spine as it lengthens upward.

3 Inhale and sweep your arms over your head as if you're making a snow angel. (B) Exhale as you bring your arms back to your sides with the same motion.

4 Repeat five times.

> TIP: Try this at the top of a hike, while standing in line, or when you need a break from your computer!

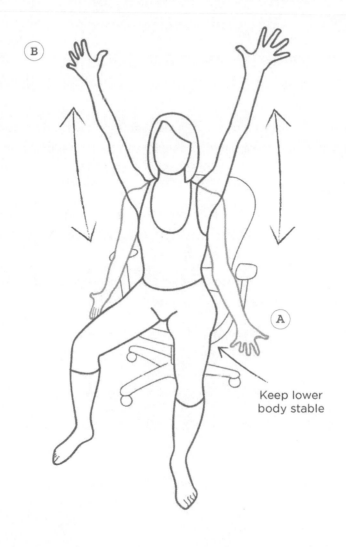

Ⓑ

Ⓐ

Keep lower
body stable

Shoulder Swing

EFFECTS Releases and awakens your shoulder joints.
EQUIPMENT None.

1 Standing with soft knees, bend your torso to the right side with your shoulders and pelvis still facing forward. Let your right arm dangle like a tassel. Place your left hand on your right clavicle, where it connects to the sternum, and feel for subtle joint movement. (A)

2 Swing your right arm back and forth (B) for about 20 seconds. Slowly let your arm come to a stop, then lift from your sternum to bring your torso upright.

3 Notice how your right side feels compared to your left side. Repeat the exercise on the left side.

> TIPS: Don't force or pull your arm into the swinging motion; instead use momentum. Avoid this exercise if you have shoulder impingement or pain.

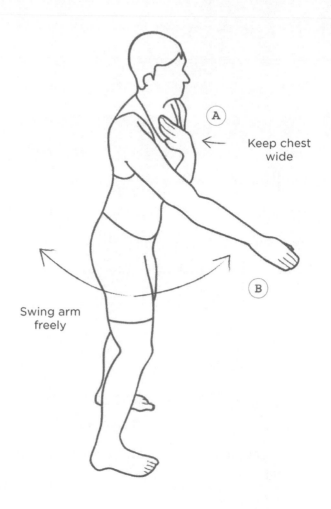

A

Keep chest wide

B

Swing arm freely

Sit, Rock, Stand

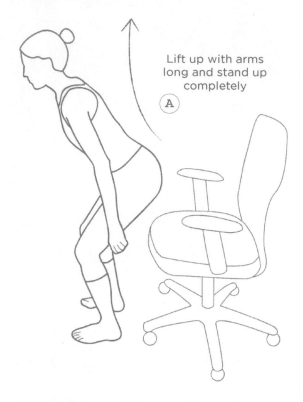

Lift up with arms long and stand up completely

Ⓐ

EFFECTS Strengthens your legs and lets you practice a neutral spine. **EQUIPMENT** A chair.

1 Start in a seated position.

2 Keeping your spine neutral, rock forward from the hips and stand up completely. Ⓐ Breathe naturally and keep your arms long by your sides.

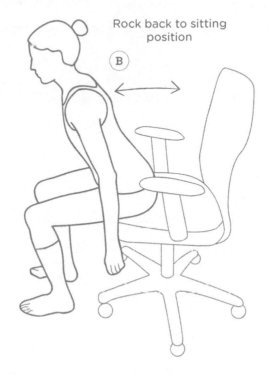

Rock back to sitting
position

B

3 To sit back down, reverse the process. Slowly lower yourself
   back into your chair, bent forward at the hips with a neutral
   spine. (B) Then rock backward from the hips until you're
   sitting up straight.

4 Repeat 10 to 15 times.

TIP: In this exercise, keep a neutral spine and lift your
body using your hips, rather than using your hands
or momentum.

Break and Shake

EFFECTS Increases your circulation, stretches your quads and hip flexors. EQUIPMENT A table for balance (optional).

1 Stand near a table to use for balance if necessary.

2 With your right hand, grab your right foot and pull it toward your glutes (A) as you press your pelvis forward and reach your tailbone toward the floor.

3 Repeat on the left side.

4 Finish by bouncing and shaking your body around for one minute to get your blood flowing.

> TIPS: Don't stick your bottom out to meet the ankle you're pulling up behind you—instead, lengthen the front of your hips. Avoid this exercise if you have knee injuries.

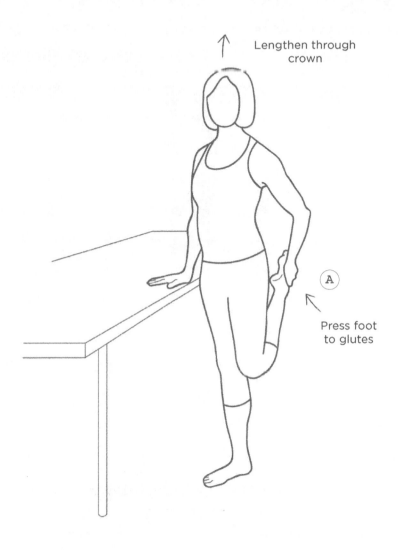

Lengthen through crown

(A)

Press foot to glutes

Eye-Directed Spine Stretch

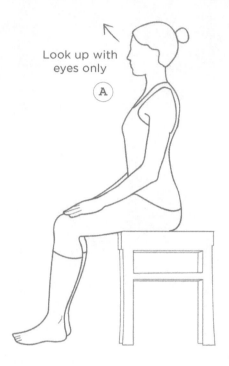

Look up with eyes only

(A)

EFFECTS Strengthens your eyes and optic nerves; develops spinal coordination, mobility, and awareness.

EQUIPMENT A chair.

1 Start in a neutral seated position with your pelvis, head, and spine in alignment, your shoulders relaxed away from your ears, and palms face down on your thighs.

2 Moving *only* your eyes, look up. (A) Slowly inhale and exhale. Then look down with eyes only. Slowly inhale and exhale. Repeat five times.

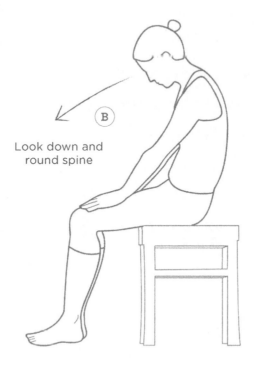

Look down and
round spine

3   For the next set, repeat the same motion, but use your spine
    along with your eyes, so that your head and torso move up
    and down as well. (B) Repeat five times, remembering to
    inhale and exhale while holding each position.

4   Return to the seated position. Moving *only* your eyes, look
    to the left, inhale, and exhale. Then look to the right, inhale,
    and exhale. Repeat five times. ▶

Eye-Directed Spine Stretch *continued*

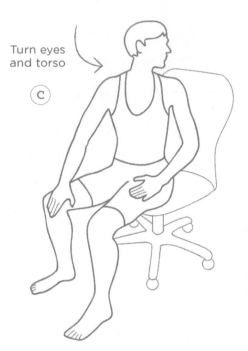

Turn eyes and torso

(C)

TIPS: Move slowly, and quit if you experience vertigo. Keep your jaw, shoulders, and breathing relaxed.

5   For the next set, repeat the same motion, but use your spine, so that your head and torso turn left to right along with your eyes. (C) Remember to inhale and exhale while holding each position. Repeat five times.

6   Return to the neutral seated postion. Look up into your eyelids and roll your eyes to the right. Inhale and exhale. Then roll them to the left. Inhale and exhale. Repeat five times.

7   Now bend your neck and torso to the right and then to the left along with your eyes, while continuing to face forward. Inhale and exhale after each motion, and repeat five times.

Seated March

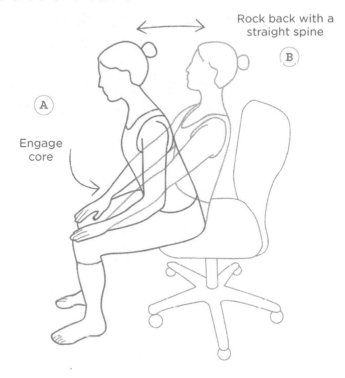

Rock back with a straight spine

B

A

Engage core

EFFECTS Promotes mental clarity, provides a posture check-in, trains your core. **EQUIPMENT** A chair.

1 Sit on the front edge of your chair. (A) Rock back and forth on your sitting bones to find your center and a strong upright posture. Hinging at the hips, rock backward with a super straight spine and engage your core. (B)

2 From this position, inhale and lift your arms overhead, then exhale and bring them back down. Repeat eight times, finishing back on your sitting bones. ▶

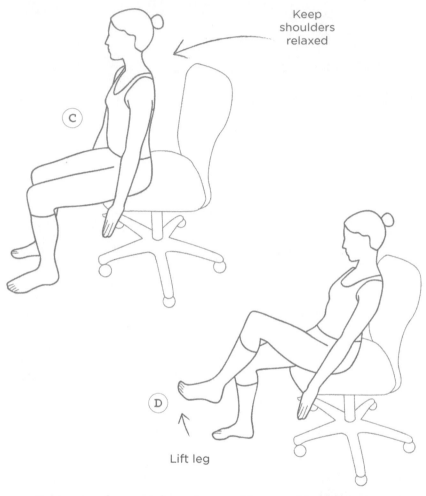

Keep shoulders relaxed

Ⓒ

Ⓓ

Lift leg

3 Return to the straight-spine position, and keep your arms at your sides. Ⓒ Hinging at the hips, rock backward. First, lift your right leg and then your left leg about 6 inches off the floor. Ⓓ Repeat eight times, using your core and keeping your arms relaxed at your sides, finishing back on your sitting bones.

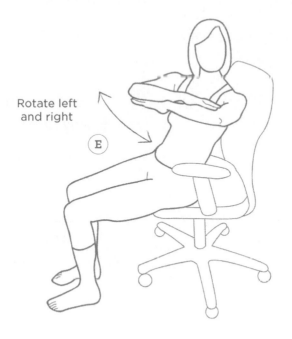

Rotate left
and right

E

4 Return to the straight-spine position, and fold your arms in front of you just below shoulder height. (E) Exhale, rock back, and rotate to the right, then inhale as you return to center. Exhale and rotate to the left, and inhale as you return to center. Repeat eight times, finishing back on your sitting bones.

TIPS: Use your legs to lengthen your spine, and keep your shoulders relaxed. Be careful not to sink into your pelvis. Avoid this exercise if you have acute back pain.

Seated Figure-Four Stretch

EFFECTS Stretches your spine, hip muscles, and glutes.
EQUIPMENT A chair.

1 Sitting as tall as you can in a chair, cross your legs by placing your left ankle over your right knee and letting your left knee fall open to the side. (A) Your legs should resemble the number four.

2 Hinging at the hip, pitch your neutral spine forward three inches. Take three breaths.

3 Bring your head down toward your shin, rounding your spine and tucking your tail beneath you. (B) Take three breaths.

4 Slowly roll your spine up until you're back in your starting position. (A)

5 Switch legs, and repeat.

> TIPS: Beginning with a straight spine and your ankle on your knee is important. Don't let your ankle creep up to your thigh. This can be a great exercise for sciatic nerve pain.

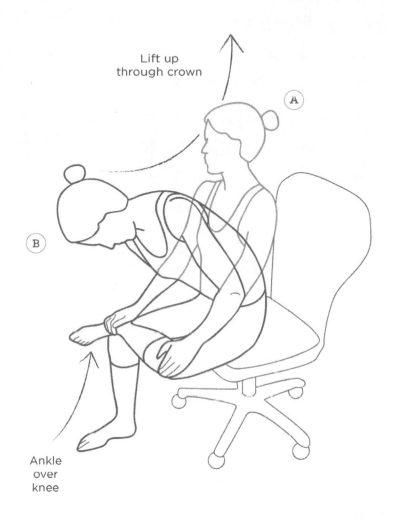

Lift up
through crown

Ⓐ

Ⓑ

Ankle
over
knee

Neck Release

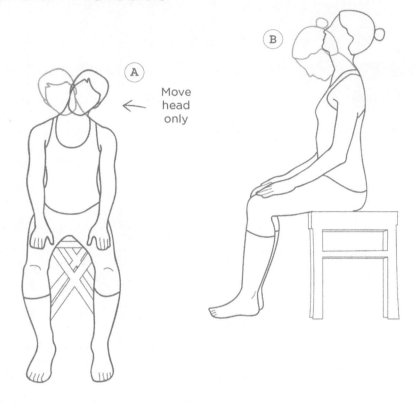

Move head only

EFFECTS Relieves neck tension, increases blood flow to your brain. EQUIPMENT A chair.

1 Start in a seated position with a neutral spine.

2 Tilt your head side to side eight times. (A)

3 Tilt your head up and down eight times. (B)

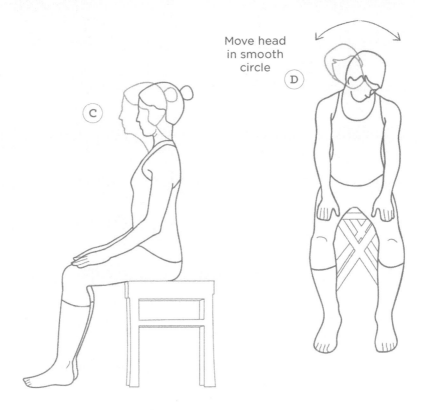

Move head in smooth circle

Ⓓ

Ⓒ

4 Push your head forward and back, like a chicken bobbing its head, eight times. Ⓒ

5 Finish by tilting your head toward one shoulder and then moving it down across your chest in a smooth half-circle to the other shoulder. Ⓓ Repeat four times, alternating sides.

TIPS: Keep your spine neutral, and move only your head. This exercise can also be done seated on the floor or standing, but a chair is recommended for helping you maintain proper posture.

Against-the-Wall Hip Stretch

EFFECTS Strengthens your glutes, improves your balance, enhances pelvic stability. EQUIPMENT A wall.

1 Stand with your right side to a wall. Lift your right leg to a 90-degree angle, knee bent, and place it against the wall. Keep your spine neutral.

2 Sink into your left hip, and then, drawing your abs in tight and reaching your head toward the ceiling, lift up out of the left hip as much as possible and press your right ankle into the wall. (A) Hold that position for a count of 10.

3 Relax to the standing position, then repeat twice more.

4 Repeat the whole process on your left side.

> TIP: Keep your body lifted and energized.

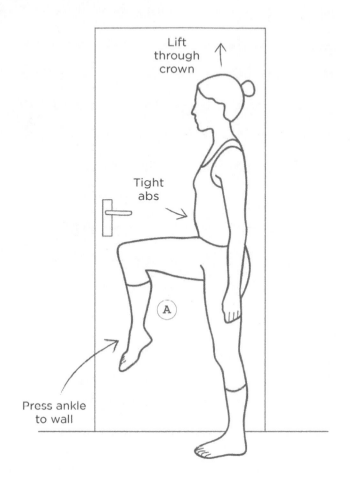

Lift
through
crown

Tight
abs

A

Press ankle
to wall

Hand and Wrist Stretch

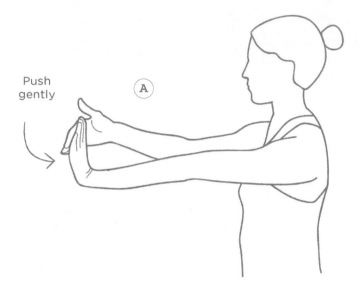

Push gently

(A)

EFFECTS Aligns and stretches your wrists; strengthens and stretches your forearms. **EQUIPMENT** None.

1 Start by interlacing your fingers and gently massaging each hand by pressing your thumb into your palm.

2 Separate your hands and reach your left arm straight out in front of you. Use your right hand to gently push your left hand backward in a flexed position, drawing the back of your hand toward the top of your forearm. (A) Hold for a count of 10.

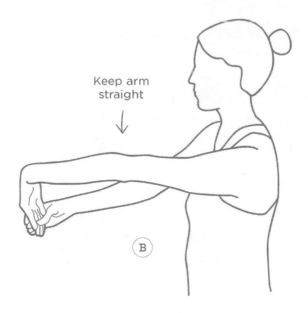

Keep arm
straight

B

3 Now gently push your left hand forward in an extended position, drawing the palm of your hand toward the bottom of your forearm. (B) Hold for a count of 10.

4 Switch hands, and repeat.

5 Finish by circling your wrists a few times in both directions.

TIP: Be gentle, and don't overstretch your wrists.

Sweeping Spinal Rotation

EFFECTS Rotates your spine, improves your coordination.
EQUIPMENT None.

1 Standing with your feet about shoulder-width apart, cross your arms in front of you just below shoulder height. Soften your knees.

2 Inhale and visualize yourself getting taller as you rotate your spine from above your waist to the right side, keeping your pelvis facing straight ahead, and arms crossed. (A) Exhale and return to center.

3 Repeat on the left. Perform three full sets.

4 Finish by releasing your arms and letting them swing naturally as you gently rotate your spine from right to left. (B)

> TIP: Avoid this exercise if you have spinal disc injuries.

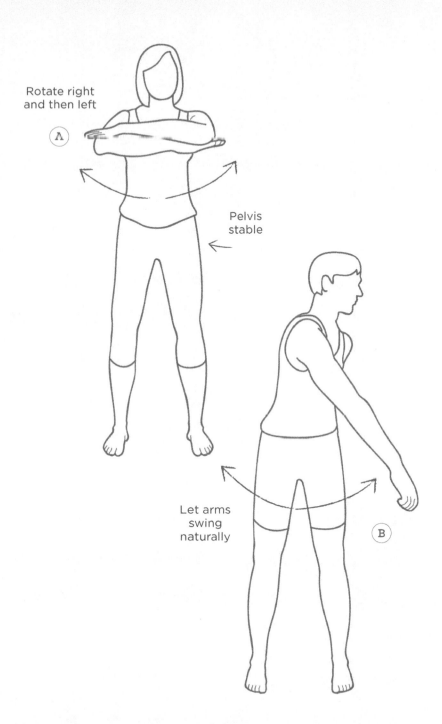

Rotate right
and then left

Ⓐ

Pelvis
stable

Let arms
swing
naturally

Ⓑ

End-of-Day Chest Stretch

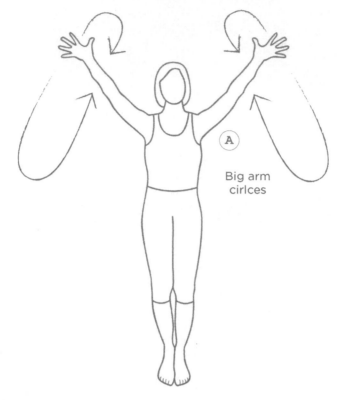

A

Big arm
cirlces

EFFECTS Opens your chest and rib cage after a long day at a desk. EQUIPMENT None.

1 In a standing position, lift your shoulders up to your ears and relax them back down.

2 Roll your shoulders up, around, and back five times, breathing deeply.

3 Inhale, spread your arms wide, and make big arm circles. (A) Exhale and release them back down, expanding your chest. Repeat five times.

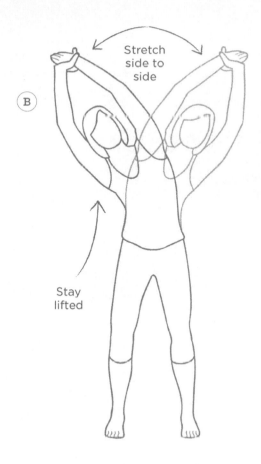

Stretch
side to
side

B

Stay
lifted

4   Place your feet shoulder width apart. Reach up toward the
    ceiling. Grab your left wrist with your right hand, stretch
    your torso laterally to the right, and hold for two deep
    breaths. (B) Then switch wrists, stretch to the left, and hold
    for two deep breaths.

> TIPS: Stay lifted. If certain ranges of motion cause
> pain in your shoulders, just do shoulder rolls or whatever
> is comfortable.

CHAPTER 5

On-the-Go Exercises

Taking your body on the road for work or pleasure doesn't mean you leave your posture exercises behind. This chapter will teach you new ways to improve your posture while traveling, exploring, or even just standing in line. Bring these on-the-go exercises with you everywhere to stay energized and aligned wherever your adventures take you.

Sunlight
Stretch

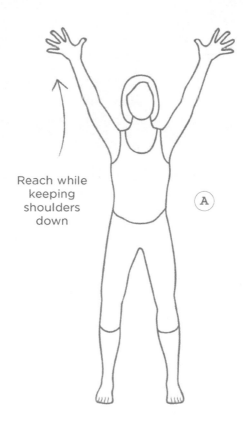

Reach while
keeping
shoulders
down

A

EFFECTS Aligns and stretches your body, helps you adjust your internal clock to a new time zone. EQUIPMENT None.

1   Stand outside facing the sun with your eyes closed.

2   Inhale and bring your attention to the space between your eyebrows. Exhale and soften this area. Inhale again and imagine this area absorbing sunlight. Exhale and imagine sending the light down your spine and legs into the earth. Do this three to five times.

3   Inhale and draw your arms overhead, stretching them toward the sky while keeping your shoulders down. (A) ▶

Sunlight Stretch *continued*

Long strong
arms

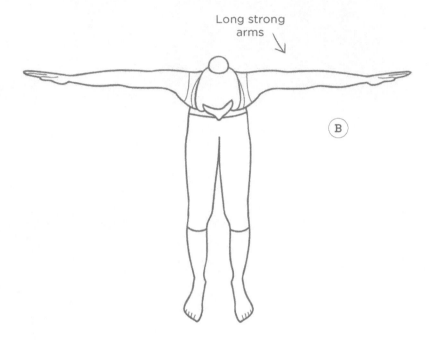

4 Exhale and fold forward from your hips as you bring
your arms out (B) and down toward your feet in a toe-
touching position. (C) (Reach for your shins if your back
or hamstrings feel tight.)

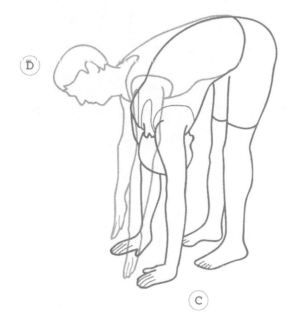

5 Inhale, look up, and extend your spine so that your torso is closer to parallel with the ground. (D) Then exhale and return to the forward fold. (C) Repeat 3 times.

6 Soften your knees, and slowly roll up through your pelvis, spine, shoulders, and head.

> **TIPS:** This is a great way to help your body get used to a new time zone. Remember to hinge from your hips and keep your shoulders relaxed.

Behind the Wheel Stretch

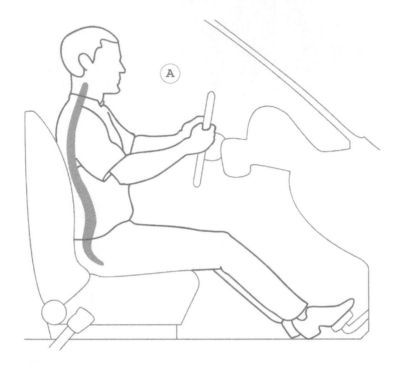

EFFECTS Enhances your circulation, increases your postural awareness while driving. EQUIPMENT A car.

1   Sit in your car seat as discussed on page 30. Your knees should be level with or a few degrees lower than your hips, your weight should be equally distributed between your sitting bones, and your spine should stay long, with a pillow or other form of lumbar support behind your lower back if necessary. Ⓐ

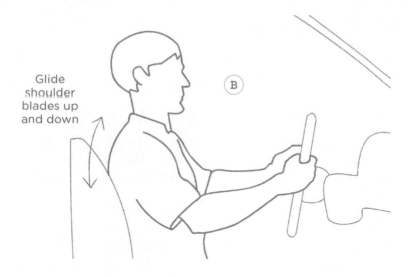

Glide shoulder blades up and down

B

2 Breathe into the back and sides of your rib cage, feeling it expand against your car seat. Exhale without letting your ribs splay forward. Repeat five times.

3 Glide your shoulders up and down five times, sliding your shoulder blades toward your back. (B)

4 Circle your shoulders five times to the front and five times to the back.

5 Engage the backs of your legs by contracting your hamstrings, and lengthen your spine for three breaths.

> TIP: You can do this stretch while driving at any time, but do make sure to stop your car for a more thorough stretch when you need one.

V-Leg Wall Stretch

EFFECTS Stretches your hamstrings, decompresses your spine, alleviates swollen ankles. EQUIPMENT A wall, a mat (optional), and a small pillow or folded towel.

1 Lie flat on your back on a mat with your legs resting against a wall at a 90-degree angle. (A) Place a folded-up towel or small pillow under your bottom against the wall. Relax there and breathe for at least one minute.

2 Slowly open your legs into a V and breathe as you stretch your lower back and open up your hips. (B) Hold for at least one minute.

> TIPS: If your legs aren't comfortable, try scooting a little farther away from the wall. This exercise is great after a long day of travel.

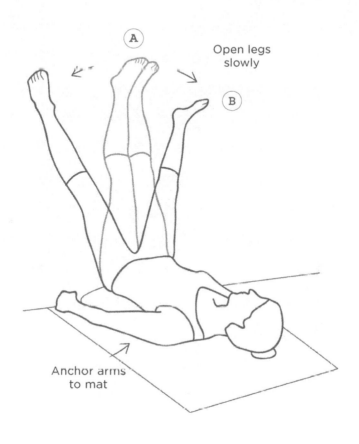

A

Open legs
slowly

B

Anchor arms
to mat

Couch Dip

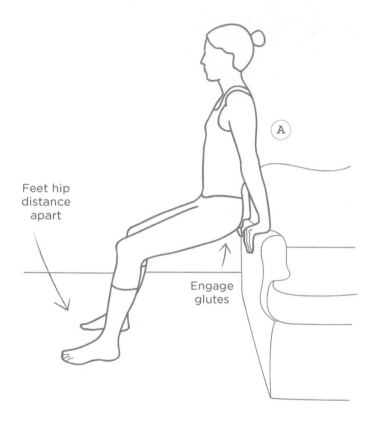

Feet hip distance apart

Engage glutes

A

EFFECTS Strengthens your triceps and shoulder girdle.
EQUIPMENT A sturdy couch or bench.

1 Sit on the arm of a couch or at the end of a bench, facing away from it with your feet hip-distance apart on the floor. Place your hands on the edge, shoulder-distance apart, and palms down with your fingers facing forward.

2 Engage your glutes, and lift yourself up off the couch arm so that you're hovering just above it. (A)

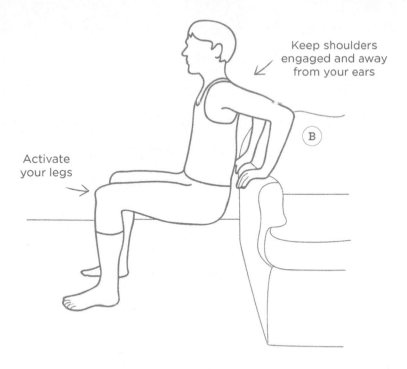

Keep shoulders engaged and away from your ears

Activate your legs

B

3 Inhale, bend your elbows, and lower your weight down past the edge of the couch for a count of four. (B)

4 Exhale and straighten your elbows, lifting yourself back up for four counts. (A)

5 Repeat 10 times, keeping your chest open and your focus straight ahead.

TIPS: Let your legs do some of the work so you're not putting too much pressure on your wrists. Keep your shoulders relaxed but stable, and don't hyperextend your elbows when you straighten them. Avoid this exercise if you have shoulder or wrist injuries.

Airplane Stretch

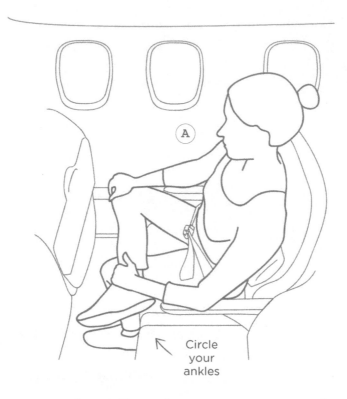

(A)

Circle your ankles

EFFECTS Stretches stiff muscles; improves your circulation; makes you more comfortable while in an airplane, train, or other cramped space. EQUIPMENT A small pillow or other form of lower-back support.

1   Bring a small pillow or other form of lumbar support on the plane with you, and put it behind your lower back.

2   Cross your ankle over your knee. (A) Circle your ankle a few times, then trace the ABCs with your toes. Switch sides, and repeat.

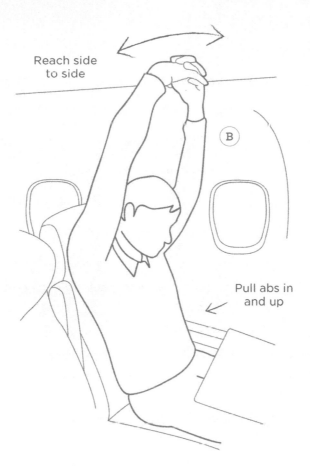

Reach side
to side

B

Pull abs in
and up

3 Interlace your fingers, and reach your hands overhead to
   decompress your spine. Keeping your pelvis stable and your
   fingers interlaced above your head, reach your arms to the
   left and then to the right. (B)

TIP: Get out of your seat, move around, and stretch as
often as possible, especially on long trips.

Plank

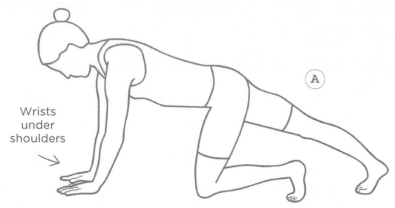

Wrists under shoulders

EFFECTS Engages your entire body, especially your core and shoulders. **EQUIPMENT** A mat.

1 Start on all fours on a mat with your wrists directly under your shoulders and your knees directly under your hips. Spread your fingers, and distribute your weight evenly through your hands.

2 Press away from the floor as you engage your back and chest muscles to stabilize your shoulders.

3 Straighten one leg (A) and then the other out behind you into a plank position, as if you were about to do a push-up. (B) Push your pubic bone slightly forward, so you're not arching your back.

4 Hold for three to five deep breaths.

5 Then, bend your elbows and place them, along with your forearms, on the mat. Keep your spine and legs in a straight line. (C)

6 Hold for three to five deep breaths, and come back to the starting position on all fours.

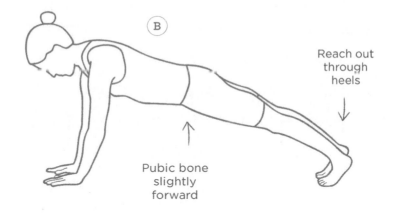

B

Reach out
through
heels

↓

↑

Pubic bone
slightly
forward

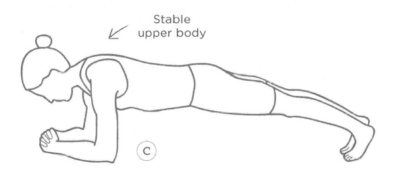

Stable
↙ upper body

C

TIPS: Keep your pelvis and head lifted and in line with
your spine. Avoid this exercise if you have wrist injuries or
acute back pain.

Wall Tap

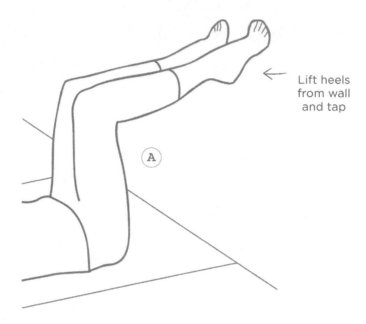

← Lift heels from wall and tap

EFFECTS Strengthens and aligns your feet and ankles.
EQUIPMENT A mat (optional), a wall.

1 Lie on your back on a mat with your hips and knees at a 90-degree angle. Press your feet into the wall, hip-distance apart.

2 Slowly lift your heels from the wall, shifting pressure to your toes, (A) all the while keeping your ankles from rolling outward or collapsing inward. From this position, tap your heels against the wall 20 times.

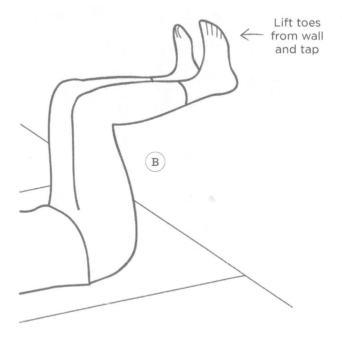

Lift toes
from wall
and tap

B

3 Now press your heels into the wall and lift your toes. (B)
From the position, tap your toes against the wall 20 times.

TIPS: Keep your feet up on the wall and your legs energized. Avoid this exercise if you have any fractured or
broken bones in your ankles or feet.

Tabletop Toe Tap

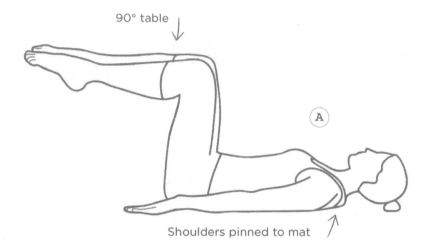

90° table

A

Shoulders pinned to mat

EFFECTS Strengthens your core, mobilizes your hip joints.
EQUIPMENT A mat.

1 Lie on your back on a mat with your knees bent and your feet on the ground hip-distance apart.

2 Inhale and engage your core. Exhale and, keeping your knee bent at a 90-degree angle, bring your right leg up until your hip also forms a 90-degree angle. Your leg is now in a table-top position. Do this four times on the right, then four times on the left.

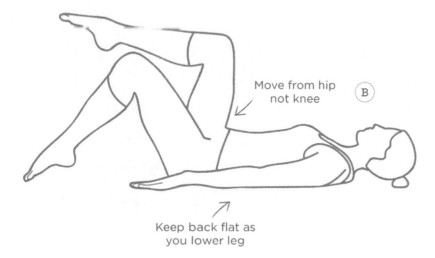

Move from hip not knee (B)

Keep back flat as you lower leg

3   Now bring both legs up to the tabletop position simultane-ously, keeping your spine neutral. (A)

4   Moving from your hip rather than from your knee, lower your left leg as far as you can while keeping your pelvis flat on the ground, then bring it back up, as if you were dipping your toes. (B) Repeat 10 times with each leg.

TIPS: Make sure your hips and knees are at 90 degrees in tabletop position and that you're moving from the hip rather than the knee. Don't stick out your belly or arch your lower back, especially when lowering your legs.

Sideways Knee Drift

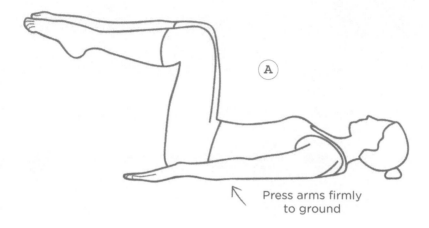

Press arms firmly
to ground

EFFECTS Strengthens your core, rotates your lower spine, enhances your shoulder and rib-cage stability.

EQUIPMENT A mat.

1 Maintaining a neutral spine, lie on your back on a mat in tabletop position—legs together in the air, hips and knees both bent at a 90-degree angle. (A) Press your arms firmly into the ground, lengthening the back of your neck and keeping your jaw relaxed.

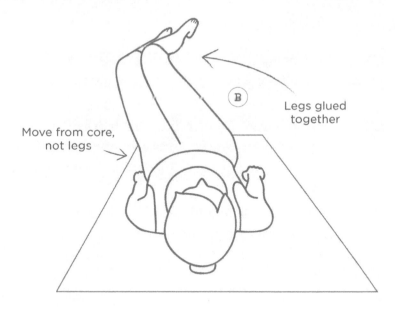

Move from core,
not legs

Legs glued
together

(B)

2 Inhale and let your legs drift together to the left. (B)

3 Exhale, engage the core muscles on the right side of your body, and bring your legs back to center.

4 Repeat five times on each side.

TIPS: Don't rotate too far to one side. You always want to be moving from your core, not your legs.

Frog Extension

EFFECTS Strengthens your lower abs and back, increases pelvic stability and hip mobility. EQUIPMENT A mat.

1 Maintaining a neutral spine, lie on your back on a mat in tabletop position—legs together in the air, hips and knees both bent at a 90-degree angle. Press your arms firmly into the ground, lengthening the back of your neck and keeping your jaw relaxed.

2 Turn your knees out slightly so that they are about a foot apart from each other. As you do so, keep your heels touching but keep your toes pointed away from each other, like a frog. (A)

3 Visualize a perfect line extending from your knees through your heels and beyond. Keeping heels together, inhale and extend your legs three inches away from the body along that line.

4 Exhale, engage your lower abs, and draw your legs back along the line into the frog position.

5 Repeat five to eight times.

TIPS: Keep your legs parallel to the ground the whole exercise. Make sure to use your core, not your legs, especially on the return motion.

Extend legs out
and draw in

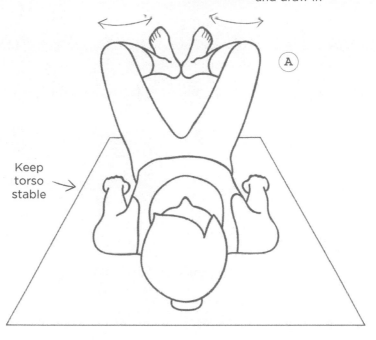

Ⓐ

Keep
torso
stable

Tourist Stretch

EFFECTS Stretches your calves and hamstrings, decompresses your spine. EQUIPMENT None.

1   From a neutral standing position, extend your left leg straight out in front of you. Flex your ankle, lifting your toes back toward your shin with your heel on the ground.

2   Bend your right knee, and shift your pelvis backward as if sitting in a chair. (A) Hinge from your hip as you fold forward as far as you comfortably can with an elongated spine, (B) stopping when you feel a nice stretch in the back of your left leg.

3   Hold for three deep breaths, then repeat the whole sequence on the other side.

> TIPS: Bend from your hips, not from your waist. Keep your neck soft, not tense.

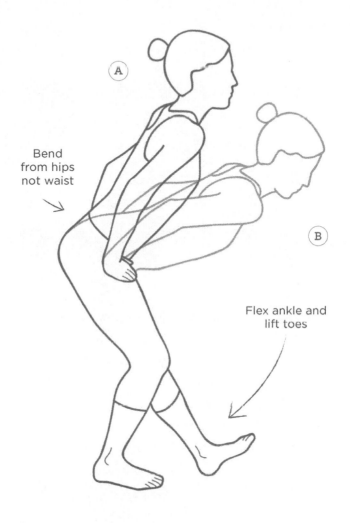

Ⓐ

Bend
from hips
not waist

Ⓑ

Flex ankle and
lift toes

Supine Knee Sway

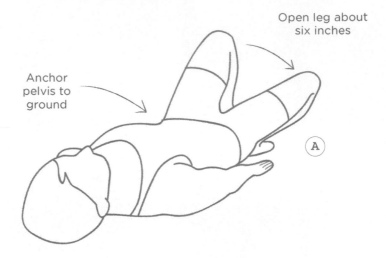

Open leg about
six inches

Anchor
pelvis to
ground

(A)

EFFECTS Strengthens your core, stabilizes your pelvis.
EQUIPMENT A mat.

1 Lie on your back on a mat with your knees bent, your feet
flat on the floor, and your legs together.

2 Inhale as you open your right leg out and down, drawing
your knee toward the floor creating about a six inch opening
while your entire pelvis stays anchored on the ground. (A)

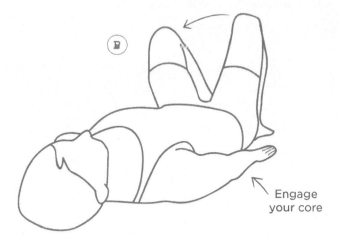

Engage
your core

3   Exhale as you engage the core muscles on the left side of
    your body to bring your right leg back to center.

4   Alternate with the left leg, (B) doing five reps on each side.

TIP: Don't let your leg open too far or your pelvis will
start to lift off the ground.

Rest Stop Stretch

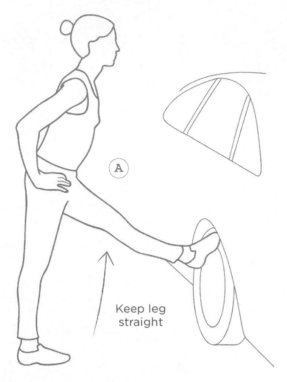

Keep leg straight

EFFECTS Stretches and aligns your body, improves your circulation. EQUIPMENT A curb, car tire, bumper, or other elevated surface.

1 Get out of your car and stretch your arms overhead, drawing your ribs away from your pelvis and decompressing your spine. Briskly walk around for at least two minutes while swinging your arms up and down.

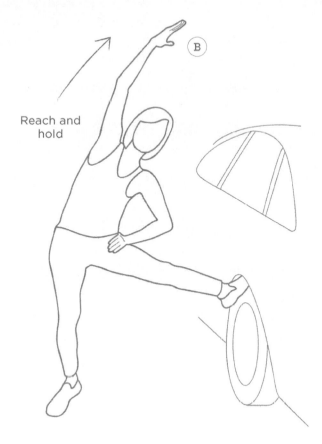

Reach and hold

2 Stand facing a car tire, bumper, or other elevated surface. Place the sole of your left foot on the surface, keeping your leg straight and your foot flexed. (A) Hinge forward at the hips as you bring your nose toward your knee. Hold for three deep breaths.

3 Keeping your left foot on the car tire, turn 90 degrees to the right so that your foot and the tire are now to your side instead of in front of you. Reach your right arm up and over your head (B) as you stretch sideways to the left, bringing your left ear toward your left knee. Hold for three deep breaths. ▶

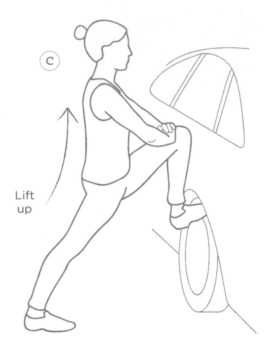

4 Keeping your foot elevated, turn 90 degrees back to the left so that you're facing the car tire again. Bend your left knee, and lean into your elevated leg, ⓒ feeling the stretch in your hip and calf. Hold for three deep breaths.

5 Repeat the whole sequence on your right leg.

> **TIPS:** Choose a surface at a height that lets you balance easily. Keep you spine and core engaged and energized.

CHAPTER 6

Healthy Posture Practices

A little bit of posture practice every day adds up to a lifetime of healthy, pain-free movement. But sometimes you just need a quick fix to help you get back on track. This chapter will offer you short-term pointers as well as exercise regimens to help you make long-term improvements to your posture.

9 to 5

Working at a desk five days a week can wear down your body if you aren't mindful. If you repeat the same unhealthy patterns daily, you'll find yourself in pain sooner than later. Start making your work environment a healthier place for you with these tips and exercises.

AGGRAVATORS: Sitting for more than an hour without getting up and moving around, slouching in your chair, bad workspace ergonomics.

QUICK FIX: Use alarms to remind yourself to get up and walk around every hour. Mix things up and try out a standing desk.

LASTING FIX: Three times throughout your workday, take 10 minutes to do the following exercises. (Even better: Do all the exercises in chapter 4 on a daily basis.)

- Snow Angels (page 82)
- Seated March (page 93)
- Sit, Rock, Stand (page 86)
- Break and Shake (page 88)

Pregnancy

Your posture changes during pregnancy, and not just because the weight of the growing fetus puts a strain on your alignment. The hormone *relaxin* softens your ligaments and joints, sometimes causing pelvic instability. You have less space in your thoracic cavity (the area holding your heart and lungs), which also means less space for your diaphragm. A conscious movement practice will carry you through your pregnancy with maximum comfort and postural alignment. Check in with your doctor before performing any new movements.

AGGRAVATORS: Relaxed ligaments, extra weight, limited space for your organs, difficulty breathing.

QUICK FIX: The cat-cow (page 59) is a great stretch for your back. Focus on breathing and hugging your baby with your abs during the "cow" portion. Gently extend into the "cat" portion, making sure it feels good.

LASTING FIX: Take 15 minutes to do the following exercises.

- Cat-Cow, Bird Dog Sequence (page 59)
- Shoulder Swing (page 84)
- Shoulder-Stretching Sequence (page 76)
- Supine Knee Sway (page 132) (Lie on a wedge pillow.)
- Clam Sequence (page 64)
- Arm-Toning Sequence (page 78)
- Seated Figure-Four Stretch (page 96)

Athletes

Athletes spend a lot of time performing the same motions over and over again, which can create wear and tear as well as postural imbalance. Use these tips and exercises to stretch out unbalanced or overworked muscle groups and get your structure aligned. You'll improve your posture *and* your athletic performance.

AGGRAVATORS: Repetitive movements that use the same muscle patterns over and over, like cycling and surfing; one-sided activities like golf, tennis, and bowling.

QUICK FIX: Work and/or stretch the underused muscle groups that tend to stay weak and/or tight. For example, when cycling, your spine rounds forward and your chest stays narrow. Counteract that form with stretches where you curve your spine backward and open your chest. For one-sided sports, perform the main movement pattern on the non-dominant side as part of a warm-up.

LASTING FIX: Take 15 minutes to warm up, stretch, and strengthen before and after your sport with these exercises.

- Shoulder-Stretching Sequence (page 76)
- Kitchen Counter Stretch (page 54)
- Supine Hamstring Stretch (page 62)
- Against-the-Wall Hip Stretch (page 100)
- Plank (page 120)
- Spinal Roll-Up (page 68)
- Couch Dip (page 116)

Over 60

To keep your body agile and strong as you mature, work on balance, alignment, and flexibility (as well as nutrition, regular exercise, and good sleep). It's easy to let discomfort stop you from moving, but that just leads to more discomfort in a vicious cycle. Healthy posture goes hand in hand with an active lifestyle.

AGGRAVATORS: Getting stuck in routines of unhealthy movement patterns, not moving consciously, getting discouraged and believing age prevents you from improving your posture.

QUICK FIX: There is no quick fix for age. Integrate the concepts of this book into your daily activities. Make your health a top priority.

LASTING FIX: Take 10 minutes every day to brush up on your balance and flexibility with the following exercises.

- Two-Minute Toothbrush Warm-Up (page 48)
- Pelvic Clock (page 52)
- Supine Hamstring Stretch (page 62)
- Cat-Cow, Bird Dog Sequence (page 59)
- Upper-Body Floor Twist (page 74)

Stress

Our body reacts to good and bad stress the same way—with muscle tension and higher cortisol levels that make healthy posture harder. No matter what's causing you stress, carve out a few minutes each day to practice these movements and keep your body feeling good.

AGGRAVATORS: Insufficient sleep, poor nutrition, commuting, deadlines, and much, much more.

QUICK FIX: Get out in nature with bare feet, and perform deep breathing exercises.

LASTING FIX: Take 10 minutes and do the following exercises when you feel stressed out and need relief.

- Wake-Up Stretch (page 45)
- V-Leg Wall Stretch (page 114)
- Sunlight Stretch (page 109)
- Tennis Ball Foot Massage (page 72)
- End-of-Day Chest Stretch (page 106)

Slumped Standing

Your standing posture is one of the first things that others notice about you. How you hold yourself affects how you engage with the world. If you practice slouching all day while sitting at a desk, your standing posture will reflect that as well. Use these exercises to stand upright with balance, ease, and confidence.

AGGRAVATORS: Being tall, having large breasts, lacking self-confidence, sitting and slouching all day.

QUICK FIX: When you notice yourself slumping while standing, align your pelvis over your feet, soften your knees, open your chest, and relax your shoulders away from your ears.

LASTING FIX: Reinforce upright standing throughout your day with these exercises.

- Shower Stretch (page 50)
- Sweeping Spinal Rotation (page 104)
- Shoulder-Stretching Sequence (page 76)
- Against-the-Wall Hip Stretch (page 100)
- Break and Shake (page 88)
- Indoor Swim (page 66)

Slouched Sitting

Your posture conforms to the environment around you. For many of us, that means hunching over computer screens, steering wheels, meals, and more. The unfortunate result is rounded shoulders, a collapsed spine, and compressed joints. Practice these exercises to learn how to sit with healthy alignment.

AGGRAVATORS: Sitting too much, without awareness, for long periods of time.

QUICK FIX: When you notice yourself slouching, stand up and move around.

LASTING FIX: Take six minutes three times a day while sitting to train your body not to slouch with these exercises.

- Snow Angels (page 82)
- Sit, Rock, Stand (page 86)
- Shoulder-Stretching Sequence (page 76)
- Seated March (page 93)
- End-of-Day Chest Stretch (page 106)

Forward-Hanging Head

Every inch your head juts forward in misalignment adds 10 extra pounds of pressure to your spine. This creates muscle imbalance, headaches, and shoulder tension. This posture is especially common for people who sit in front of a computer all day.

AGGRAVATORS: Leaning forward when using computers, phones, and tablets; studying and reading; commuting.

QUICK FIX: When your head starts to slide forward, stack your pelvis, chest, and head, and reach through the crown of your head. Keep your jaw and shoulders relaxed. Use your eyes to gaze around instead of your entire head and neck.

LASTING FIX: Keep your head aligned in just a few minutes each day with the following exercises.

- Neck Release (page 98)
- Eye-Directed Spine Stretch (page 90)
- Snow Angels (page 82)
- Shoulder Swing (page 84)

Stiff Neck

Whether you slept on it funny or simply stared at a screen for too many hours in a row, a stiff neck can negatively affect your entire day. It inhibits your movement, throws off your alignment, and even causes headaches. Remedy the situation as soon as you can with these posture fixes.

AGGRAVATORS: Poor posture and head placement throughout your day, shoulder tension, stress, sleeping in a position in which your head and neck aren't supported properly.

QUICK FIX: Gently massage your neck to get some blood flowing and release some tension. Get a pillow that supports your neck while you sleep.

LASTING FIX: Take five minutes to stretch your neck and release tension three times a day with these exercises.

- Neck Release (page 98)
- Eye-Directed Spine Stretch (page 90)
- Airplane Stretch (page 118)

Uneven Shoulders

It's not uncommon for one of your shoulders to be higher than the other. Many people overuse their dominant side during daily activities like writing, carrying bags, or lifting-up young children. No one's body is perfectly symmetrical, but you do want to look out for postural imbalance. These exercises will help balance your shoulders.

AGGRAVATORS: Overuse of one side of your body, scoliosis or other abnormal spinal curves, stress.

QUICK FIX: Notice where your shoulders live on your rib cage, and make subtle adjustments by breathing into your rib cage. Create length in your spine, and shift your ribs to the side of your lower shoulder. But don't overcorrect—you'll just create more tension.

LASTING FIX: Level out your shoulders by doing these exercises for 10 minutes throughout your day.

- Snow Angels (page 82)
- Neck Release (page 98)
- Shoulder Swing (page 84)
- Shoulder-Stretching Sequence (page 76)
- Upper-Body Floor Twist (page 74)

Flabby Stomach

It can be frustrating when you eat well and work out regularly yet still have a belly, but some of that overhang has more to do with your posture than your fitness level. Add these exercises to get your core back in action so you're not pushing your tummy out any farther than you need to.

AGGRAVATORS: Poor diet, sitting too much, lack of abdominal muscle tone.

QUICK FIX: Finding your natural, neutral posture will immediately reduce the pooch.

LASTING FIX: Spend 15 minutes a day with these exercises. Focus on drawing your navel in toward your spine.

- Pelvic Clock (page 52)
- Spinal Roll-Up (page 68)
- Tabletop Toe Tap (page 124)
- Supine Knee Sway (page 132)
- Sideways Knee Drift (page 126)
- Frog Extension (page 128)
- Plank (page 120)

Rounded Shoulders

If your posture is unbalanced, you may be using your neck, back, or chest to do work your shoulders should be doing. This lets your shoulders become weak and rounded. Luckily, it's a relatively easy problem to fix. Practice these movements to rediscover your shoulders, open your chest, and bring ease to your neck and spine.

AGGRAVATORS: Hunching in front of a computer, having large breasts, trying to hide your height.

QUICK FIX: When you realize your shoulders are rounding forward, draw them down while opening across your collarbones and sternum, and rotate your arms outward.

LASTING FIX: Practice these exercises 10 minutes every day.

- End-of-Day Chest Stretch (page 106)
- Shoulder-Stretching Sequence (page 76)
- Couch Dip (page 116)
- Indoor Swim (page 66)
- Upper-Body Floor Twist (page 74)

Lower-Back Pain

Although studies indicate that 60 to 80 percent of adults will experience chronic back pain at some point, you don't have to be one of them. By learning how to strengthen your back muscles, mobilize your spinal joints, and distribute force equally through your entire spine, you can improve your posture and live pain-free.

AGGRAVATORS: Sitting too much, sitting in the same position for too long, having weak muscles in your hips and glutes and along your spine, overusing some spinal movements and underusing others.

QUICK FIX: To help relieve lower-back pain, take some deep breaths into the area that hurts to soften and release the tension. If possible, gently go through the Pelvic Clock sequence (page 50). And schedule a massage, acupuncture, or chiropractor appointment!

LASTING FIX: Take 12 minutes each day to warm up, stretch, and strengthen your back.

- Pelvic Clock (page 52)
- Pelvic Curl Sequence (page 70)
- Indoor Swim (page 66)
- Cat-Cow, Bird Dog Sequence (page 59)
- Airplane Stretch (page 118)
- Eye-Directed Spine Stretch (page 90)

Misaligned Feet and Ankles

The human foot has 26 bones, 33 joints, 107 ligaments, and 19 muscles and tendons. That's a lot of opportunities for something to get out of whack! And your feet are the foundation of your entire body, so imbalance there often causes imbalance all the way up. Follow these tips for grounded, well-supported feet.

AGGRAVATORS: Wearing flip-flops, high heels, or any shoes that lack support; having knees or ankles that rotate too far inward or outward.

QUICK FIX: Kick your shoes off, sit down, and rub your feet.

LASTING FIX: Take 10 minutes a day to give your feet some attention.

- Wall Tap (page 122)
- Two-Minute Toothbrush Warm-Up (page 48)
- Tennis Ball Foot Massage (page 72)

References

American Academy of Pain Medicine. "AAPM Facts and Figures on Pain." Accessed November 30, 2015. www.painmed.org /patientcenter/facts_on_pain.aspx.

American Chiropractic Association. "Back Pain Facts & Statistics." Accessed November 30, 2015. www.acatoday.org/Patients/ Health-Wellness-Information/Back-Pain-Facts-and-Statistics

Cleveland Clinic. "Diaphragmatic Breathing." Accessed November 30, 2015. my.clevelandclinic.org/health/diseases_conditions/hic _Understanding_COPD/hic_Pulmonary_Rehabilitation_Is_it _for_You/hic_Diaphragmatic_Breathing.

Cuda, Gretchen. "Just Breathe: Body Has a Built-In Stress Reliever." NPR. Last modified July 15, 2011. www.npr.org/2010/12/06/131734718 /just-breathe-body-has-a-built-in-stress-reliever.

Dalton, Sarah. "Breathe Deeper to Improve Health and Posture." Healthline. October 23, 2013. www.healthline.com/health /breathe-deeper-improve-health-and-posture#1.

Lipton, Bruce. *The Biology of Belief: Unleashing the Power of Consciousness, Matter & Miracles.* Carlsbad, CA: Hay House, Inc., 2005.

Park, Alice. "Sitting is Killing You." *Time.* September 2, 2014. time.com/sitting.

Reynolds, Gretchen. "Sit Less, Live Longer?" *New York Times.* September 17, 2014. well.blogs.nytimes.com/2014/09/17/sit-less-live-longer/.

Resources

BOOKS

8 Steps to a Pain-Free Back: Natural Posture Solutions for Pain in the Back, Neck, Shoulder, Hip, Knee, and Foot by Esther Gokhale

Anatomy Trains: Myofascial Meridians for Manual and Movement Therapists by Tom Myers

Atlas of Human Anatomy by Frank Netter

Natural Posture for Pain-Free Living: The Practice of Mindful Alignment by Kathleen Porter

WEBSITES

Alexander Technique—www.alexandertechnique.com

Anatomy Trains—www.anatomytrains.com

The Feldenkrais Method—www.feldenkrais.com

Foundation Training—www.foundationtraining.com

Franklin Method—www.franklinmethodonline.com

Gokhale Method—gokhalemethod.com

GYROTONIC® Expansion System—www.Gyrotonic.com

Lumo Lift Postural Device—www.lumobodytech.com/lumo-lift

Mayo Clinic—www.mayoclinic.org

Nia Technique—www.Nianow.com

Pilates Studio City—www.PilatesStudioCity.com

Index

Acknowledgments

LORA My heart fills with love and gratitude for all the support I have in my life. I will never be able to acknowledge all the beautiful people who have made this book possible, but here are a few. My mom and dad, who believed in my dream to be a dancer and sent me off into the world with confidence. My daughter, Lola, who keeps me on my toes and fills my days with pure joy. My friend Amy Dickerson, who connected Nikki and me to this project and keeps cheering me on. My marvelous movement and dance teachers for sharing all your wisdom with me and teaching me grace. My best friend and business partner, Nikki, for collaborating with me on this adventure and making every moment transformative. My husband, Jim, my love, who keeps me laughing and learning and said "go for it."

NIKKI I am filled with deep gratitude for the friends, clients, and family who have blessed my life with their love and support. Thank you for always encouraging me and letting my visionary spirit soar. Thank you to my many mentors and teachers who have pioneered new movement and healing disciplines. You have taught me to be present to the human experience, to embody flow with dynamic ease, and to be a more effective teacher. Thank you to Sanda Thompson for helping me continue to deepen, grow, and transform, and for your beautiful example of the creative art of living. To my best friend and business partner, Lora, for all of our adventures and for your endless love and inspiration. To my husband, Keith, who makes me laugh and loves me in all of my quirkiness. You have taught me how to honor my health and wild creativity with dimensionality and courage.

About the Authors

LORA PAVILACK Lora is a former professional dancer who has performed around the world, including as a Radio City Rockette. With Nikki Alstedter, she co-owns Pilates Studio City in Southern California and Pilates South Austin in Texas. She is a Master Teacher in Pilates through the Pilates Sports Center and is certified in Gyrotonic, Gyrokinesis, the Franklin Method, and Da Vinci BodyBoard, among other body-balancing disciplines. Her mission is to help people improve their posture, strength, and balance through movement so they can stand tall and enjoy life to the fullest.

NIKKI ALSTEDTER Nikki is a former dancer, choreographer, and aerial acrobat who has performed in Los Angeles, Japan, and across Europe. She is the founder of Arlùnviji Transformative Movement in Santa Barbara, and she co-owns, with Lora Pavilack, Pilates Studio City in Southern California and Pilates South Austin in Texas. A student of the energetic healing system Quantum Kinetics, she has two decades of experience helping clients participate in life with greater physical ease and awareness. She currently teaches Gyrotonic, Gyrokinesis, Pilates, Da Vinci BodyBoard, Nia, and the Franklin Method and is a Master Teacher for Pilates Sports Center and the Da Vinci BodyBoard system.

9 781623 157180